Eating for Sport

SHELLY MELTZER AND CECILY FULLER

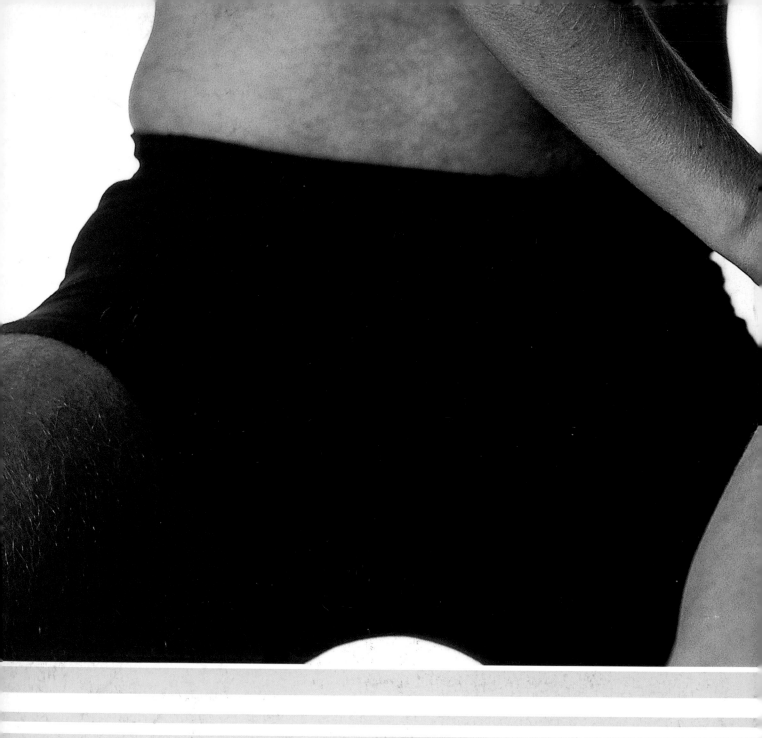

NH
NEW
HOLLAND

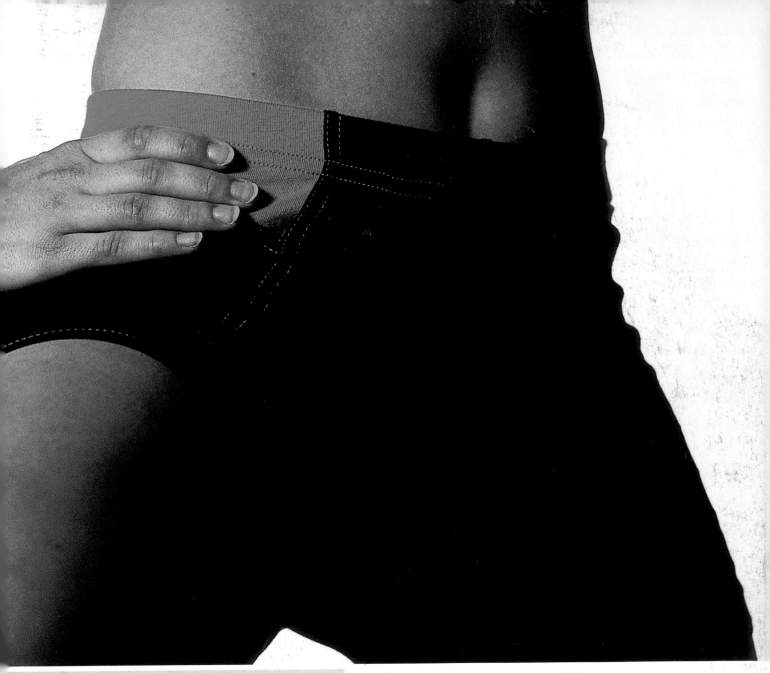

Eating for Sport

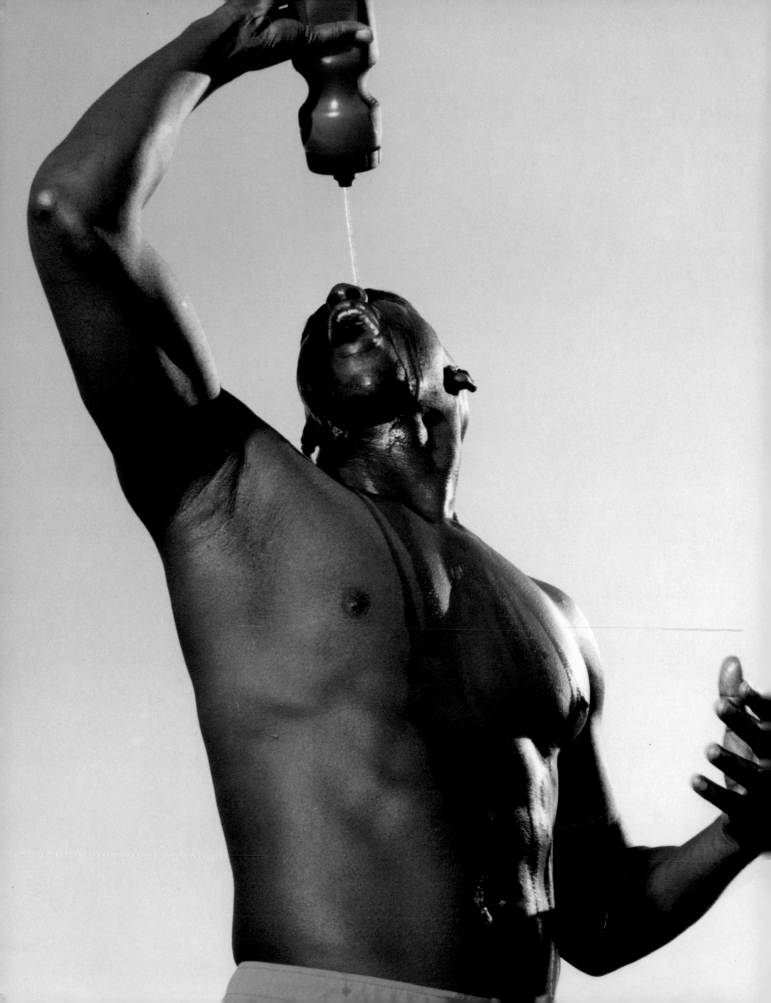

To Craig, Benjamin and Kira Meltzer
and Norman and Elizabeth Fuller

First published in 2005 by New Holland Publishers

London ∎ Cape Town ∎ Sydney ∎ Auckland

www.newhollandpublishers.com

86 Edgware Rd	80 McKenzie St	14 Aquatic Drive	218 Lake Road
London	Cape Town	Frenchs Forest	Northcote
W2 2EA	8001	NSW 2086	Auckland
United Kingdom	South Africa	Australia	New Zealand

ISBN 1 84330 859 2 (HB)

ISBN 1 84537 081 3 (PB)

PUBLISHING MANAGERS Claudia dos Santos & Simon Pooley

COMMISSIONING EDITOR Alfred LeMaitre

PUBLISHER Mariëlle Renssen

EDITOR Anna Tanneberger

DESIGNER Nathalie Scott

ILLUSTRATOR Steven Felmore

PICTURE RESEARCHER Tamlyn McGeean

PROOFREADER Leizel Brown

PRODUCTION Myrna Collins

CONSULTANT Dr Adam Collins
Nutrition lecturer, British College of Osteopathic Medicine

Reproduction by Resolution Colour Pty Ltd, Cape Town

Printed and bound in Malaysia by Times Offset (M) Sdn Bhd

1 3 5 7 9 10 8 6 4 2

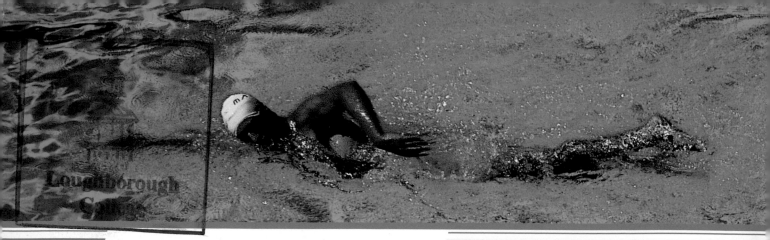

contents

Part 1
Nutrition basics and nutritional needs

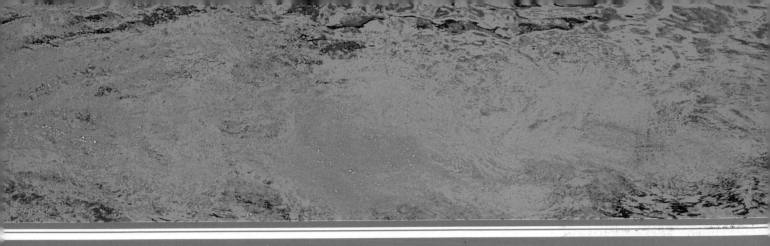

Part 2
Sport-specific nutrition

Each section outlines the physical demands and characteristics of a group of sports with common nutritional issues.
Case studies highlight common problems and how they can be solved.

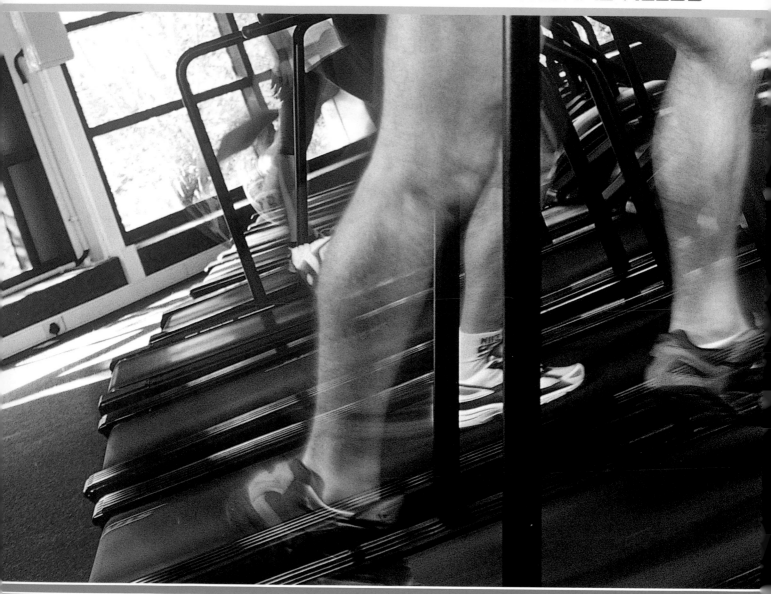

Introduction

MYTHS, FACTS AND SCIENCE

IT IS THROUGH MANY YEARS of combined experience and having the unique privilege of working at the Sport Science Institute of South Africa that this book has evolved. We have worked with many general fitness enthusiasts, development, elite and Olympic athletes as well as international teams, and so have been able to develop a comprehensive hands-on nutritional approach, which integrates cutting-edge scientific principles that will help all individuals, regardless of their level of sport, to achieve their common goal – to perform at their best.

Sports nutrition is no longer a secret, based solely on anecdotal evidence. Before the 1960s, sports nutrition had evolved largely through self-experimentation, trial and error, and tradition, but with relatively few controlled studies. Sports nutrition is now a well-established science in its own right and it is well recognized that diet affects an athlete in many ways.

At the very basic level, good nutrition plays an important role in the maintenance of health, allowing the athlete to train and compete. Understandably an athlete needs to be healthy, and free of injury and illness to train adequately. Beyond health maintenance, nutrition can have a serious effect on performance through hydration, weight maintenance, and providing optimal fuel to train, compete and recover repeatedly.

Nutrition is a controllable factor that plays a role through the entire life of an individual; and for a world-class athlete proper nutrition can make the difference in winning, assuming that all other factors (genetic, behavioural, socio-economic, cultural and environmental) are equal.

Sportspersons are constantly bombarded with the latest sports nutrition fashions and trends. Too often, the magic offered by sports supplements diverts attention away from real performance enhancing and controllable factors like sports-specific nutrition matched to training regimes. It is a challenge to keep abreast and make practical sense of all this information, to separate the facts from the myths, and then to incorporate this into training and competition routines.

This book consolidates the scientific research in such a way that the athlete, the parent, the trainer, the clinician and dietitian are provided with practical and sport-specific nutrition game plans. Recommendations take into account the real life situations in which athletes find themselves and the foods that are most likely to be available to them. At times this means recommending the best choice of fast foods, for instance. To get the most out of this book, read part 1, which gives a good overview of sports nutrition and introduces new concepts such as fat-loading, the latest modified fluid guidelines, new issues around chronic fatigue, travel and jet lag, male eating disorders as well as the use and abuse of some of the latest supplements. Part 2 divides sports (ranging from golf, gymnastics, weightlifting, running, rowing, and team sports to extreme sports) into different chapters, depending on the features of each sport that affect nutrition requirements.

MEASUREMENTS

We tried to give quantities in user-friendly measurements. Amounts were rounded off to be more practical. Metric quantities were converted to measurements most commonly in use for that particular food. No conversions were given where the metric measurement is the international standard, for instance in scientific formulae and Olympic distances. The mathematical symbol ≈ is used to indicate the approximate equivalent.

NUTRIENTS

When we refer to a nutrient (carbohydrate, protein, fat or alcohol), it is always in g (grams).
Examples: 50g carbohydrate list
1.5–2g protein/kg body weight
500g carbohydrate per day
(Micronutrient requirement expressed as a percentage of daily intake can be misleading due to the wide range of requirements of athletes in different sports. It is also more practical and direct to give grams of nutrient per kilogram of body weight.)

ENERGY

Both kilojoules (kJ) and kilocalories (kcal) are provided.
1kcal = 4.82kJ, 1kJ = 0.2389kcal
When referring to the unspecified energy content of food or a person's energy intake in general, we used the word 'calories', which seems to be understood worldwide. In this book the word 'calories' refers to kilocalories (kcal).

RECOMMENDED DIETARY ALLOWANCES

Dietary Reference Intakes (DRIs) consist of four different values: Estimated Average Requirements (EAR), Recommended Dietary Allowances (RDA), Adequate Intakes (AI), and Tolerable Upper Intake Levels (UL).

In the United Kingdom, however, Dietary Reference Values (DRV) are used. It is the generic term for Estimated Average Requirement (EAR), Reference Nutrient Intake (RNI) and Lower Reference Nutrient Intake (LRNI).

European Union regulations require Recommended Daily Amounts (RDAs) to be shown on food and supplement labels.

These recommendations are rough estimates and are always open to debate.

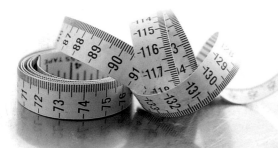

WEIGHT/HEIGHT

Kilograms (pounds) and metres (feet and inches)

1kg = 2.205 lb, 1m = 3.281ft

FOOD QUANTITIES [SOLIDS]

Household measures were chosen

250ml = 1 cup

25ml = 2tbsp

5ml = 1tsp

Ounces were chosen for smaller quantities, e.g. 90g (3 oz)

1g = 0,05327 oz

Pounds were chosen for larger quantities, e.g. 250g (½ lb)

1kg (1000g) = 2.205 lb

Other practical quantities were left as is e.g. 2 sports bars, 3 medium fruit.

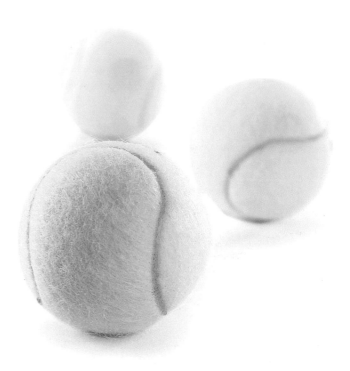

FLUID QUANTITIES

Metric measurements have been converted into the measurement most commonly used for that particular fluid. Since most quantities are estimates and rounded off, we made no effort to distinguish between the UK and US measurements where these differ.

Water and sports drinks were converted to pints

(1 litre = 2.11 US pints or 1.76 UK pints)

Fruit juice to fluid ounces

(1 litre = 33.814 fl oz US and 35.195 fl oz UK)

Colddrink quantities were converted from ml to fl oz.

Quantities of milk, yoghurt and liquid meal replacement were converted to cups.

ALTITUDE

Metres to feet (1m = 3.281ft)

DISTANCE

Metres to yards (1m = 1.094yd), but note that Olympic distances were kept as standard.

SIZING IT UP

ONE SERVING	SIZE-WISE
90g (3 oz) red meat/poultry/fish	Deck of playing cards
Medium apple/pear 150g (5 oz)	Tennis ball
30g (1 oz) cheese	One matchbox
125ml (½ cup) of ice cream	Tennis ball
125ml (½ cup) of pasta/rice/vegetables	Tennis ball
30g (1 oz) or 2tbsp nuts/sweets	one handful
1 medium potato (90g; 3 oz)	Computer mouse
1 biscuit (15g; ½ oz)	A bath plug
250ml (1 cup) of cereal	A tight fist
5ml (1tsp) butter	A thumb tip
1 muffin/cinnamon bun/roll	A doorknob or fist
1 pancake or waffle	A CD

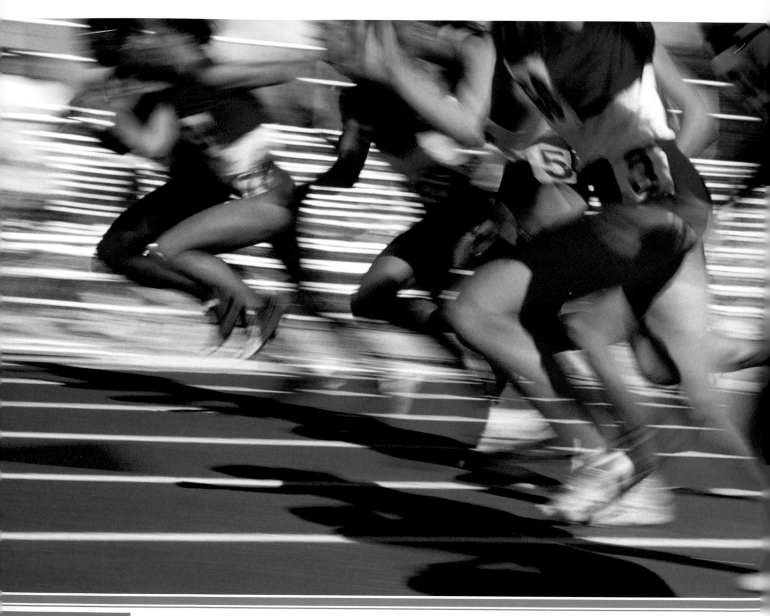

chapter 1

FROM FOOD TO FUEL

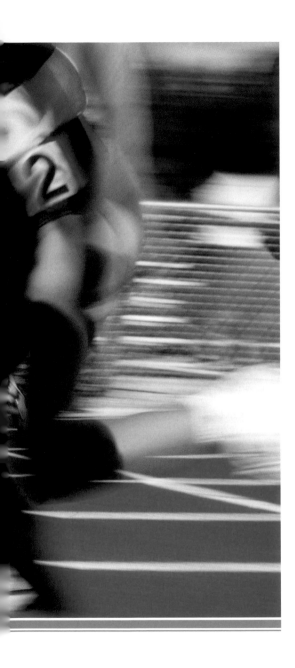

THE CONTRIBUTION OF NUTRITION TO PERFORMANCE

The belief that nutrition plays an important role in physical fitness goes back to ancient times when athletes and soldiers preparing for battle consumed certain foods such as lion heart and deer liver for increased agility, speed or strength. Eating fashions of athletes have changed and, with the advancement of scientific methods (for instance, muscle biopsy techniques) and nutritional technologies, deer liver and lion heart have been replaced by substances such as carbohydrate powders, amino acids, creatine, sodium bicarbonate, amino acids and l-carnitine. However, in their quest for optimal performance, the underlying belief in the ergogenic – or performance-enhancing – abilities of certain foods and nutrients by athletes and fitness enthusiasts has remained the same.

Clearly, a fundamental role of nutrition in sport is to supply fuel for energy as well as all the essential nutrients and fluid. However, there is currently much debate on the bigger role that nutrition may play in enhancing performance by decreasing the perception of effort. There are also specific stressors that nutrition may counteract in sportspersons of different ages, genders and health status (see p33).

There has been a dramatic increase in the number of nutritional supplements on the market, all packaged with promises and claims of addressing one or more of the performance-limiting factors highlighted in the illustration on page 14.

In most cases nutrition and supplement recommendations are made without scientific evidence or taking into consideration how these recommendations will affect the athlete's overall diet. Scientifically controlled studies to determine the effects of nutrition on sporting performance are costly and complex. There are also other factors that affect performance such as genetics, sleep, rest, training, skills, mental attitude and equipment.

Sports nutrition also has a practical role to play in advising on strategies to overcome problems such as limited time available for food preparation, travel nutrition or lack of appetite before a match. With a good understanding of the nutritional content and functions of food, sports supplements and fluid, as well as the energy demands of a sport, you can manipulate your diet to improve endurance, aid recovery, alter your body composition (muscle-to-fat-mass ratio), reduce fatigue, and improve mental performance and skill.

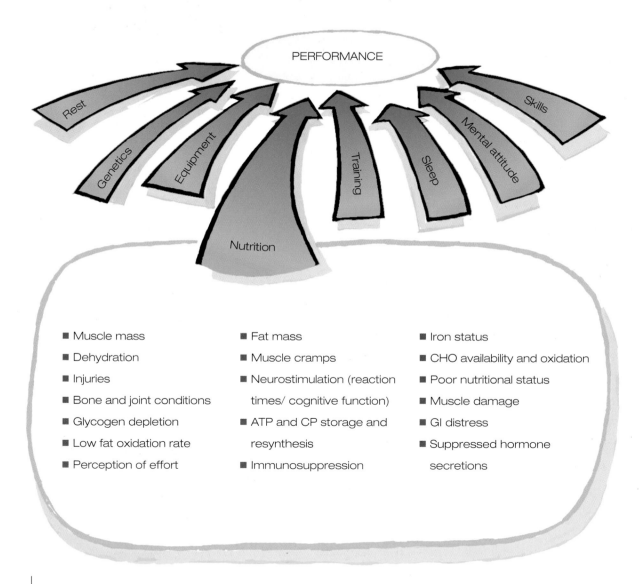

- Muscle mass
- Dehydration
- Injuries
- Bone and joint conditions
- Glycogen depletion
- Low fat oxidation rate
- Perception of effort

- Fat mass
- Muscle cramps
- Neurostimulation (reaction times/ cognitive function)
- ATP and CP storage and resynthesis
- Immunosuppression

- Iron status
- CHO availability and oxidation
- Poor nutritional status
- Muscle damage
- GI distress
- Suppressed hormone secretions

Above *The role of nutrition and the components of performance.*

CHO = carbohydrate

ATP = adenosine triphosphate

CP = creatine phosphate

GI = gastrointestinal

THE SUPPLY OF ENERGY

ENERGY SOURCES FROM THE DIET

Energy, measured in kilojoules or kilocalories (1kcal = 4.18kJ), is provided by the macronutrients carbohydrate, protein and fat. These nutrients are needed by the body in relatively large amounts.

CARBOHYDRATES

FUNCTION

No matter what your sport, carbohydrate (foods rich in starches and sugars, see 50g carbohydrate list p17) is the critical fuel for optimal performance. Exercising muscles rely on carbohydrate as the main source of fuel. Therefore diets low in carbohydrate can lead to a lack of energy during exercise, early fatigue, loss of concentration and delayed recovery. All carbohydrate, once digested, are eventually converted into blood glucose or stored as glycogen in the liver and muscle for later use. Excess carbohydrate will be stored as fat.

Since the 1920s scientific studies have revealed the ergogenic properties of carbohydrates. Later studies showed that a relatively high carbohydrate intake appears to delay the onset of fatigue during endurance-type events. This refers to pre-event carbo-loading of 600–700g/day to maximize liver and muscle glycogen stores. Similarly, carbohydrate ingestion during exercise also delays the onset of fatigue by sparing liver glycogen, but the mechanisms of this effect seem to be governed by central regulatory functions rather than solely as a consequence of delaying an impending 'energy crisis'.

There is also evidence that in high-intensity, intermittent exercise lasting less than one hour, carbohydrate loading and carbohydrate ingestion during exercise (30–60g/hr) appear to impart some neuro-protection from fatigue.

MACRONUTRIENT	ENERGY
Carbohydrate	17kJ/g (4kcal/g)
Protein	17kJ/g (4kcal/g)
Fat	38kJ/g (9kcal/g)
*Alcohol	29kJ/g (7kcal/g)

Above *Energy content of macronutrients. *Although alcohol supplies energy, it is not available as a source of fuel during exercise and has little nutritional value (see pp68–69).*

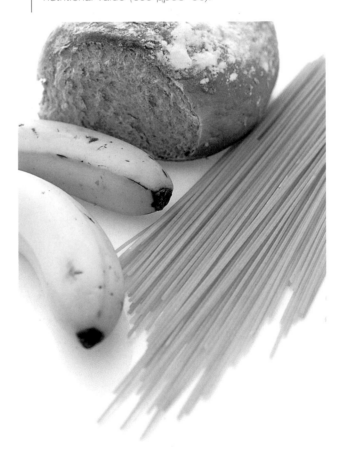

Above *In the world of performance, carbohydrates are essential. Once ingested, they are turned into glucose and stored in the muscles and liver as glycogen.*

In summary, all the evidence shows that carbohydrates have an important role before, during and after exercise. This may vary between individuals and the mechanisms are not completely understood. Ingesting carbohydrate during exercise is the most effective way of preventing hypoglycaemia (low blood sugar levels).

STORES

The total amount of carbohydrate that your body can store as glycogen in the liver and muscle is minimal (about 600g; 1.3 lb) compared to your body's fat stores. Liver glycogen stores are used to top up the glucose levels in the blood to ensure that the brain maintains its essential glucose supply. Regular training rapidly depletes these small reserves and you therefore need to ensure an adequate daily carbohydrate intake. Decreasing glycogen stores can cause your body to start breaking down muscle protein for much-needed glucose. This will have unfavourable consequences, one of which is the loss of lean muscle mass, and therefore strength.

FOOD SOURCES

Carbohydrate-rich foods include grains, cereals, dairy produce, fruit, certain vegetables, sports-specific products and sugar. The amount you need depends on your training programme and other dietary goals. Your training requirements will be in the range of 5–7g/kg body weight, with a maximum of 600–700g per day (60% of energy intake, or more). However, this may vary depending on your daily energy expenditure, type of sport, gender and environment. In situations involving either extremely prolonged and intense exercise or repeated bouts within an 8–12 hour period, requirements may increase to 8–10g/kg body weight. In extreme sports such as the Tour de France, this may be as high as 12g/kg body weight (*see p168*). For weight loss, carbohydrate intake may be reduced to 3–4g/kg body weight.

Every plate of food you eat should contain at least 50% carbohydrate-rich foods (*see p23*). First determine your total daily carbohydrate requirements in grams, then divide that figure by 50, for the number of carbohydrate servings needed per day. Then select the appropriate number of items from the list of 50g carbohydrate servings (*see opposite*).

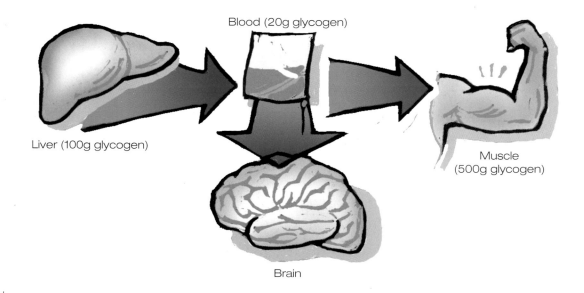

Blood (20g glycogen)

Liver (100g glycogen)

Muscle (500g glycogen)

Brain

Above *Carbohydrate is stored in the liver and muscle as glycogen. The liver glycogen is broken down to glucose and released into the bloodstream to ensure a constant supply to the brain and muscle.*

GRAINS
1 CUP = 250ML (9 OZ)

- 3 thick slices bread
- 10 crackers or 6 rice cakes
- 500ml (2 cups) high-fibre (bran) cereal
- 3 breakfast wheat biscuits
- 500ml (2 cups) porridge
- 250ml (1 cup) pasta or 1 heaped cup rice
- 250ml (1 cup) samp/polenta/couscous
- 3 medium bran muffins
- 2–3 muesli or breakfast bars

VEGETABLES & LEGUMES
- 250ml (1 cup) baked beans
- 830ml (3⅓ cups) peas; or carrots; or butternut; or mixed vegetables
- 3 medium potatoes; or 250ml (1 cup) sweet potato (270g; ¼ lb)

FRUIT
- 3 medium pieces of fruit (apple, banana)
- 40ml (3½tbsp) raisins
- 500ml (17 fl oz) fruit juice

DAIRY
- 1ℓ(4 cups) skim- or low-fat milk or buttermilk
- 375ml (1½ cups) low-fat, flavoured, drinking yoghurt or 250ml (1 cup) fruit yoghurt

SPORTS PRODUCTS, SUGARS AND SWEETS
- 60ml (5tbsp) sugar
- 1 handful of jelly babies
- 10 marshmallows (100g; 3⅓oz)
- 1–2 sports bars
- 40ml (3½tbsp) glucose polymer powder
- 1–1½ sachets gel
- 500ml (2 cups) liquid meal replacements (made with low-fat milk or water)
- 800–1000ml (1½–2pt) sports drinks
- 500ml (17 fl oz) cola or other soft drink

Practical tips

1. Enjoy a variety of carbohydrate-rich foods to optimize your nutrient intake, focusing on nutrient-dense carbohydrates that are also rich in vitamins, minerals and fibre (wholegrain cereals, fruit and vegetables).

2. Split your total carbohydrate needs into several meals and snacks throughout the day.

3. Always have portable choices such as fruit, yoghurt, sports bars and dried fruit on hand.

4. Carbohydrate-rich foods are sometimes classified according to the speed at which they are absorbed from the blood. This is referred to as the glycaemic index (GI). High GI, carbohydrate-rich foods are absorbed more quickly (sports drinks, energy bars, bread and jam) and are therefore good choices after exercising.

5. If you have little appetite and/or suffer from stomach discomfort (for instance, before exercising), then compact, easily digestible carbohydrate foods should be eaten – sweetened, low-fibre breakfast cereals, white bread with honey or jam, or sugar. Carbohydrate glucose polymer powders can be added to foods and drinks to boost your carbohydrate intake. Liquid meal supplements can also be used.

6. Decrease your carbohydrate intake when your training decreases (for instance, in the off-season or when injured) to prevent unnecessary weight gain.

7. Sports drinks can help you meet your daily carbohydrate needs, but not as a main source of carbohydrate, because this will reduce your vitamin, mineral and fibre intake and may lead to weight gain.

Left *List of 50g carbohydrate servings from which to make up your total daily requirement.*

FAT

FUNCTIONS

Fat is the most concentrated form of energy, providing double the amount of kilojoules (calories) as an equal amount of carbohydrate or protein (*see p15*). However, it is not a readily available source of energy during exercise. Even when you exercise at a low to moderate intensity, fat, because of its slow rate of utilization, can only provide about 50% of the energy needed – the other 50% still comes from carbohydrate. Furthermore, dietary fat is easily stored as fat in the body. It is only in rare situations that fat has a positive effect on performance. A fat-loading regime (*see p176*) may be of benefit prior to participating in an ultra-endurance event that would challenge the muscle glycogen stores. Carrying extra body fat can be an advantage in certain sports: in open water long-distance swimming the extra body fat offers buoyancy and insulation; and in certain positions of play in some team sports (such as a lock or prop in rugby) it protects organs. However, in most sports, extra body fat is simply additional dead weight, affecting the athlete's speed and agility.

Eating too little fat also carries risk as fat provides fat-soluble vitamins and essential fatty acids, the latter specifically having important immune protective functions. Some fat in the diet is also needed to enhance the absorption of these nutrients and of course offers palatability.

High-fat meals or snacks are not recommended just before training or competing as they slow down the rate of stomach emptying. This means that the food remains in your stomach for longer, increasing the risk of stomach discomfort and, moreover, the fat crowds out the opportunity for much-needed carbohydrate.

In summary, in most situations, eating fat before an event is not beneficial and may be counterproductive. Only in certain events, such as polar expeditions, will fat help meet these requirements during the event. In the immediate post-exercise recovery period priority should also be given to carbohydrate and protein, keeping fat intake low.

The average lean athlete has 9–12kg (20–26 lb) of body fat and it has been estimated that this amount of stored body fat (adipose tissue) alone could supply sufficient energy for nearly four days of running. Despite these extensive fat reserves, there are still many factors that limit the body's ability to use (oxidize or burn) fat as a fuel during exercise (*see pp28, 30,148*).

Below left *'Added' fat should be limited to about a third of total daily fat allowance.*
Below right *Different levels of body fat are required for different positions of play.*
Opposite *The fat content of commonly eaten foods according to portion sizes.*

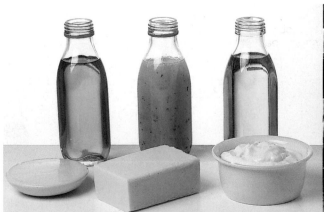

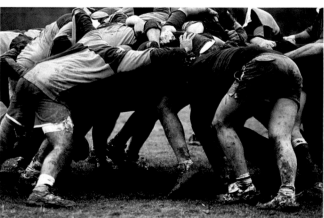

FOOD GROUP	less than 5g FAT	5–10g FAT	more than 10g FAT
MILK	250ml (1 cup) fat-free (skim) milk, 250ml fat-free yoghurt	250ml (1 cup) low-fat (2%) milk, 250ml (1 cup) low-fat yoghurt, buttermilk	250ml (1 cup) full-cream milk
ANIMAL PROTEIN IN 100G [3½ OZ] PORTIONS	Low-fat fish (hake, kingklip), calamari, crayfish, prawns/shrimps, oysters, mussels, tuna in brine, chicken breast (no skin), ostrich, venison, egg white	Snoek, salmon, pilchards, tuna in oil, chicken dark meat (no skin), lean veal, lean pork, lean beef, ham, egg yolk	Sardines in oil, fried fish, chicken with skin, mutton, sausages, polony, bacon, liver and organ meats
CHEESE	60g (2 oz) fat-free cottage cheese/Ricotta, 60g (2 oz) fat-free cream cheese, 60g (2 oz) low-fat cottage cheese, 30g (1 oz) low-fat cheese spread	30g (1 oz) low-fat Edam, 30g (1 oz) Mozzarella, 30g (1 oz) Feta	30g (1 oz) Cheddar, 30g (1 oz) Sweetmilk, 20g (½ oz) Parmesan, 60g (2 oz) low-fat cream cheese, 60g (2 oz) regular cream cheese
STARCHES (grains and cereals)	Bread, rolls, crackers, cereal, porridge, low-fat muesli, rice, pasta, potatoes, oil-free muffins	Homemade bran muffin	Pies, cakes, croissants, cake muffins
FRUIT	Fresh and dried fruit, fruit juice	¼ avocado pear	Coconut
VEGETABLES	All varieties	–	–
LEGUMES AND SOYA PRODUCTS	Portion of beans, lentils, soya mince	Portion of soya sausages and burgers	–
FATS	5ml (1tsp) extra light or light margarine, 15ml (1tbsp) low-oil and oil-free salad dressings	5ml (1tsp) regular margarine, 5ml (1tsp) butter, 10ml (2tsp) peanut butter, 5ml (1tsp) canola, olive or sunflower oil, 6 olives, 15ml (3tsp) sandwich spread	25ml (2tbsp) nuts
SUGAR & DESSERTS	Sugar, honey, syrup, jam, hard sweets, jelly babies, nougat, marshmallows, jelly, fruit sorbet, fruit lollies, low-fat frozen yoghurt, custard prepared with fat-free milk	–	50g (1.7 oz) chocolate bar, regular ice-cream, cream (dairy and and non-dairy) coffee creamers
BISCUITS	2 plain biscuits, 1 slice Swiss roll	2 biscuits with fillings, shortbread	–
SNACKS	45g (1½ oz) plain pretzels, unbuttered popcorn	45g (1½ oz) flavoured pretzels, 30g (1 oz) reduced-fat crisps	30g (1 oz) packet crisps, 30g (1 oz) cheese popcorn
OTHER	Fishpaste, yeast extracts	–	–
TAKE-AWAYS/ CONVENIENCE MEALS	Home-made pizza prepared with low-fat base with fruit and vegetable toppings	Chicken burger (no mayonnaise), spicy rice, fish burger, lean burger	Fried chicken and chips, burgers
BEVERAGES	Portion of colddrink, juices, low-fat drinking chocolate	Malted drinks prepared with low-fat milk	Milkshakes

Recent research has, however, shown how in some situations these limitations can be overcome (see p30).

Your body fat and body shape is largely determined by your genetic make-up (determined by your parents) and is something you cannot change. Dietary and training strategies can, to a certain degree, remould your body shape, but you should ultimately choose a sport that suits your natural physique best! Recommended ranges for body fat levels do exist for certain sports, but it is important to have realistic and sensible body fat goals because of the following factors:

- Maintenance of lower body fat levels might not always be sustainable, often compromising overall nutritional status because it might involve highly restrictive eating patterns.
- Very low body fat levels (below 3–5% for males and 14% for females) are associated with negative health and performance outcomes. In females this can lead to irregular or cessation of menstruation which can lead to increased bone loss and bone diseases like osteoporosis (see p76). Athletes may also experience early fatigue, intolerance to cold and have an increased risk of infection.
- Improved performance is not always associated with very low body fat levels and in fact some athletes will perform better with body fat levels above the recommended range.

FOOD SOURCES

All fat-containing foods provide a mixture of fats (saturated, mono- and polyunsaturated fats). All these fats are equally rich in calories and are easily converted and stored as body fat. There is, however, some recent evidence that the polyunsaturated fats (found in foods like sunflower oil and fatty fish) are the most easily oxidized (burnt). Therefore, when planning your 'daily fat budget' you should always give preference to polyunsaturated fats and the 'healthy' mono-unsaturated fats (found in foods like olive oil, canola oil and avocado pear and nuts) and reduce your intake of foods rich in saturated fats like fatty meat, chicken skin, coconut, full cream dairy products, lard and ghee. Another reason to limit your saturated fatty acid intake is that it increases blood cholesterol levels the most. Cholesterol is only found in foods of animal origin and, like saturated fats, should be limited because it is converted into blood cholesterol.

The total amount of fat (in grams) that you need depends on your total energy requirements, body composition goals, sport type, and other risk factors. Broadly speaking, every plate of food you eat should provide 20–30% of energy from fat, but it is important to note that some of this fat will be provided by protein (cheese, meat, chicken, fatty fish, full- and low-fat dairy foods) and what is often referred to as hidden fats in snacks and sauces (see p19).

Practical tips

1. Limit your intake of both 'added' and 'hidden' sources of fat. Butter, margarine, avocado pear, peanut butter and oil are examples of added fats, whereas hidden fats are those found in high-fat cheeses, many processed meats such as polony and salami and snack items such as chocolates, crisps and nuts.
2. Try not to double-up on fat at a meal. Choose between peanut butter, margarine or avocado pear as a spread on bread and choose either olives or salad dressing with salad.
3. Read labels to get an indication of the fat content in food and always choose the lower fat options.
4. Use low-fat cooking methods (grill with little oil, stir-fry, steam or oven-bake).
5. Vegetable sources of fat such as sunflower, olive or canola oils and spreads are healthier than hard margarine or butter.

PROTEIN

FUNCTIONS

Your body not only needs protein, it also needs a sufficient quantity of each of the amino acids, the building blocks of protein. There are 21 amino acids, nine of which are essential in the diet since the body cannot manufacture them.

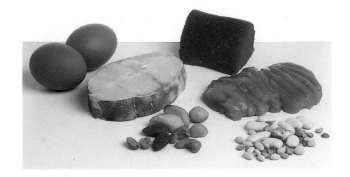

Amino acids are needed to manufacture the structural components of muscle tissue, enzymes, haemoglobin, antibodies, hormones and transport proteins. They are therefore needed for strength, to build and maintain muscle, maintain immune function, to aid recovery and, in younger athletes, protein is also essential for growth and development.

Protein is not an efficient source of fuel during exercise, but when too little energy is available from carbohydrate and fat, amino acids will be used as energy. In this situation, amino acids are broken down to form glucose and nitrogen. The nitrogen waste produced must not be allowed to accumulate in the body as it is toxic and it is therefore converted to urea and excreted from the body by the kidneys.

One of the biggest myths is that large amounts of protein are required to build muscle. Your muscles can only use a limited amount of protein for growth, provided there is enough carbohydrate to fuel the strength-training required

for your muscles to grow. Any excess protein will be broken down for energy and excreted as urea, although excessive protein intake may increase total calorie intake, increasing the chances of weight gain. The process of breaking down amino acids also necessitates the excretion of water and so excessive intakes of dietary protein may affect fluid balance. A consistently high protein intake may also contribute to kidney disease, gout and arthritis.

Above *Vary your protein intake to provide a selection of different nutrients.*
Below *There is no storage form of protein, but the body is continually synthesizing protein from the pool of amino acids within cells and then breaking them down again.*

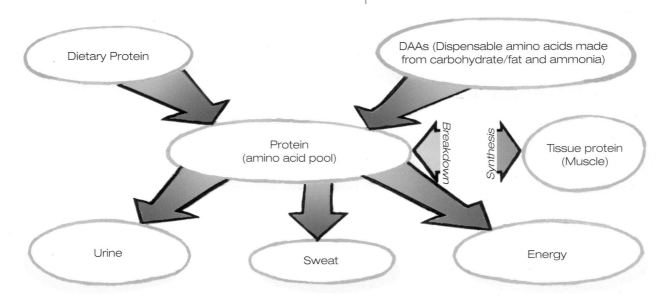

FOODS AND PORTION SIZES PROVIDING 10G PROTEIN

- 50g (1.7 oz) grilled fish (cooked)
- 50g (1.7 oz) tuna, salmon, pilchards
- 35g (1.3 oz) lean beef, lamb, veal or game (cooked)
- 40g (1.3 oz) chicken or turkey (skinless, cooked)
- 50g (1.7 oz) ostrich (cooked)
- 2 small or 1 large chicken egg
- the whites of 3 large eggs
- 70g (2.3 oz) cottage cheese
- 30g (1 oz) low-fat cheese
- 200ml (¾ cup) low-fat fruit yoghurt
- 300ml (1¼ cups) low-fat milk (cow or soy milk)
- 30ml (2tbsp) low-fat or skim milk powder
- 250ml (1 cup) liquid meal replacement (made up with skim milk or water)
- 160ml (⅔ cup) cooked lentils
- 125ml (½ cup) cooked soya beans
- 200ml (¾ cup) baked beans
- 40ml (3½tbsp) nuts*
- 60ml (5tbsp) sesame seeds
- 200ml (¾ cup) cooked soya mince
- 120g (4 oz) raw tofu
- 125ml (½ cup) hummus*
- 70g (2.3 oz) Quorn (textured vegetable protein)

* These foods have a high fat content

However, extra protein may be needed after training, a competition or match and especially so if you have experienced any muscle or tissue damage. Muscle damage also interferes with the storage of carbohydrate as glycogen, so together with the extra protein you should also increase your carbohydrate intake (*see Recovery Nutrition p55*).

Above *Foods in portion sizes of 10g protein. See the table on p11 (Sizing It Up) on how to estimate the size of portions.*

STORES

There is no storage form of protein as such, but the body is continually synthesizing protein from the pool of amino acids within cells and then breaking it down again. Unlike carbohydrate and fat stores, which can be more easily manipulated by dietary means, the amino acid pool is more tightly regulated to allow protein to be used preferentially for vital body functions other than energy. This makes the dietary manipulation of amino acid stores for muscle growth more challenging, which is probably why many athletes resort to alternative methods.

FOOD SOURCES

Current accepted recommendations on protein requirements for athletes fall in the range of 1–2.2g/kg body weight or as a percentage of total energy intake (15–20%). Protein requirements in exceptional situations such as pregnancy, high altitude and low-energy eating will be discussed later. The emphasis should always be on good quality protein of high biological value such as lean red meat, chicken, fish, eggs and low-fat dairy, which are rich in all the essential amino acids and are also the primary sources of certain micronutrients such as calcium, vitamin B_{12} and bio-available iron and zinc. A low intake of protein and poor quality protein can lead to deficiencies of these micronutrients.

Vegetable sources of protein are considered to be of low biological value since they do not provide the full range of the essential amino acids. Therefore, even if you have sufficient protein (amount in grams) but one of the essential amino acids is lacking (the limiting amino acid) you will not be able to utilize the other amino acids to synthesize protein! This should not be interpreted as an excuse to supplement with single amino acids. Safety and efficacy data is still lacking for single amino acid supplementation and so no upper safety limits have been set.

Vegetarians who eat plant foods only, in the absence of complementary mixtures of plant protein may have an inadequate intake of essential amino acids (*see pp 81, 82*).

Practical tips

1. Choose a variety of protein-rich foods.
2. Protein should also be distributed throughout the day. Do not let protein dominate all meals, so that you leave enough space on your plate for all the carbohydrate needed.
3. Always choose lean meat and low-fat dairy products as many of these protein-rich foods contain hidden sources of fat.
4. If you are a vegetarian you need to make a special effort to ensure that your diet provides enough good quality protein. By mixing different vegetable proteins such as baked beans on toast, lentils and rice, or a peanut butter sandwich you will achieve good protein combinations (*see p82*).
5. Many proteins are expensive so it is important to explore ways of extending or stretching the protein without reducing the nutritional value. Dried beans and lentils can be added to stews and soups. Other good economical sources of protein include pilchards, sardines, eggs and skim milk powder (which can be added to many drinks, cereals and soups).
6. Commercially available, specially formulated liquid meal replacements that provide carbohydrate and protein can also be used.
7. To increase your muscle mass you need to follow your eating plan and training programme. If you only concentrate on a high protein intake without enough carbohydrate, then the protein will be used for energy instead of being used to build muscle! Moreover, too little carbohydrate will lead to low energy levels, which will make it very difficult for you to train and perform at your best.

PLATE MODEL

Below is a model of what your plate should look like when you dish up your meals: carbohydrate-rich foods should cover two-thirds of your plate, while the rest (one-third) should be reserved for protein-rich foods, with a minimal amount of added fat such as butter, margarine, oil, cream or mayonnaise.

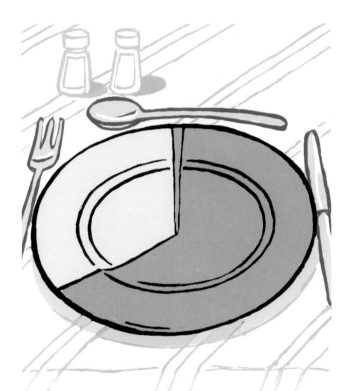

PROTEIN
Egg, fish, lean meat/chicken, low-fat dairy, legumes (beans/lentils/chickpeas), soya, tofu.

ADDED FAT
Butter, margarine, oil, mayonnaise, salad dressings, cream.

CARBOHYDRATES (CHO)
Bread, pasta/rice, corn/maize, vegetables, fruit. Moderate amounts of concentrated CHO (sugar, jam, syrup, honey, chutney, tomato sauce) can be added for flavour and to boost your CHO intake.

Above *Visualize this model when dishing up.*

VITAMINS AND MINERALS AND THEIR IMPACT ON ENERGY

Vitamins are organic compounds required in very small amounts, and a distinct feature is that the human body is unable to synthesize them. Most vitamins regulate processes essential for normal metabolism, growth and development. Those vitamins involved in energy metabolism are like the spark plugs of an engine. They do not provide energy but are involved in the production of energy from fuel stores by acting as catalysts for metabolic reactions. More specifically, they are responsible for the storage and utilization of energy in the body.

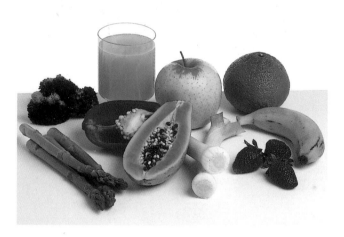

Vitamins are either classified as fat soluble (A, D, E and K) or water soluble (B complex and C). The fat-soluble vitamins are stored in body tissues, so consuming excessive amounts of these vitamins, especially vitamin A, can lead to toxicity and organ damage. Water-soluble vitamins, on the other hand, are not stored in the body and any intake in excess of daily requirements generally results in 'expensive urine'.

MICRONUTRIENT	GOOD FOOD SOURCES
VITAMINS	
Thiamin (vitamin B$_1$)	Fortified breakfast cereals, whole-wheat breads, pork, liver, legumes, nuts, yeast (vegetable) extract and brewer's yeast
Riboflavin (vitamin B$_2$)	Dairy products, red meat, fish, poultry, eggs, fortified cereals
Niacin (vitamin B$_3$)	Lean meat, chicken, fish, legumes, eggs, fortified cereals, nuts
Pyridoxine (vitamin B$_6$)	Lean red meat, poultry, fish, eggs, wholewheat breads and cereals, nuts, bananas, yeast (vegetable) extract, soya beans
Pantothenic acid	Liver, yeast, egg yolk, red meat, dried fruit, nuts
Biotin	Liver, red meat, egg yolk, nuts, peanut butter
MINERALS	
Magnesium	Wholegrain cereals, legumes, nuts, sesame seeds, dried figs, green vegetables
Iron	Organ meat, lean meat, egg yolk, dried fruit, fortified cereals, dark green leafy vegetables
Zinc	Oysters, red meat, dark meat of chicken, peanuts, sunflower seeds, wholegrain cereals, legumes
Copper	Organ meats, shellfish, nuts and seeds, mushrooms, cocoa
Chromium	Red meat, liver, egg yolk, seafood, wholegrain cereals, molasses

Above left *Eat at least five different fruit and vegetables every day.*

Above right *Vitamins and minerals needed for energy metabolism.*

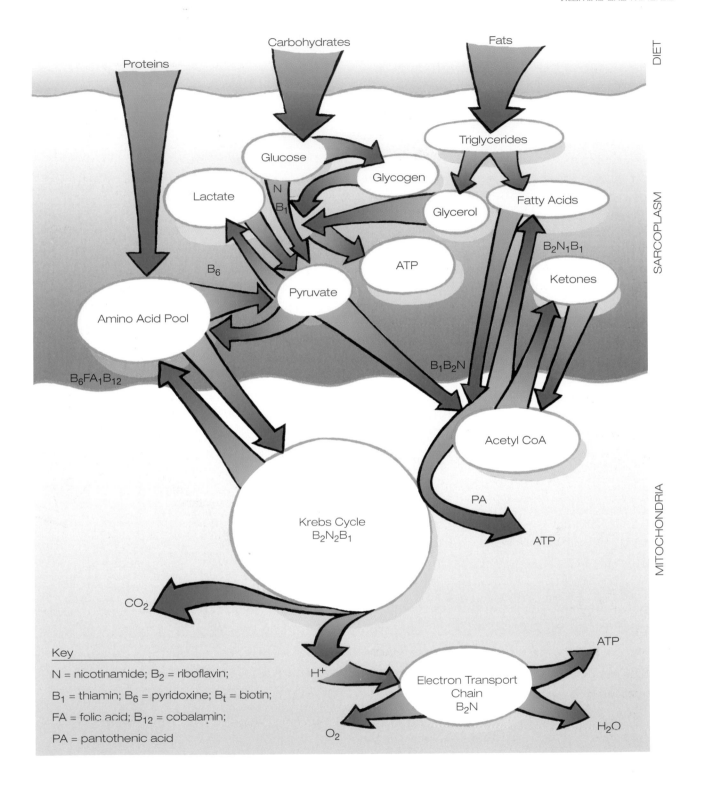

Above *The role of B complex vitamins in energy metabolism.*

Although these vitamins tend to be non-toxic, very large amounts have been found to impair the absorption and utilization of other nutrients. The most important vitamins and minerals needed for energy metabolism and production are the B Complex group, magnesium, iron, zinc, copper and chromium (*see p24*). Vitamins of the B complex group are involved with muscle contraction, nerve function, and also act as co-factors of enzymes for energy metabolism as do iron, zinc, copper and chromium. Other functions of these nutrients include haemoglobin synthesis, immune and antioxidant function, tissue repair and protein synthesis.

Deficiencies in any of these vitamins will impair metabolism, sports performance and, of course, health. Generally, athletes' diets have been shown to supply adequate vitamins and minerals, provided the diet is well planned and varied to meet the athletes' energy requirements. Those at risk are low-energy consumers, chronic carbohydrate loaders and athletes not able to meet overall nutritional needs (calcium and iron, for instance) through diet alone. Specific situations, such as exercising at altitude or in extreme environmental conditions or athletes with chronic fatigue or with special medical problems, may also have increased requirements (*see p89*). It is widely accepted that vitamin deficiencies will impair performance, but there is no evidence to show that supplementing a diet already adequate in vitamins and minerals will enhance performance. Supplementation of vitamins is discussed in more detail in chapter 7.

Practical tips

1. Correcting dietary deficiencies through food should always be the first approach, before considering supplementation, because nutrients coexist in foods. The assistance of a registered dietitian is recommended.

2. Enjoy eating a wide variety of fruits and vegetables – the more colour and crunch the better. Aim for an intake of between 5–9 fruit and vegetables per day.

3. Where possible choose fresh produce, especially those in season. Frozen vegetables, if cooked correctly, are also nutritious.

4. Limit the storage time of vegetables. Shop regularly for fresh produce and, if buying market produce, ensure that the fruit and vegetables have not been standing in the sun for any length of time.

5. Avoid overcooking. Limit the amount of water used, keep the lid on the pot and limit cooking times.

6. Do not add bicarbonate of soda to colour green vegetables as this destroys the B vitamins.

7. Make use of fortified cereals.

8. To enhance iron absorption:

   ■ When eating non-meat (eggs, whole grains and fortified cereals, lentils, soya, green leafy vegetables) sources of iron, add a food rich in vitamin C because vitamin C increases the absorption of iron. Foods rich in vitamin C include tomatoes, citrus fruit, guavas, strawberries, broccoli and green peppers.

   ■ Avoid tea or coffee with your meal as caffeine and tannin decreases iron absorption.

   ■ Remember that an iron supplement will not correct other nutritional inadequacies. If you are worried about your iron status, then have your iron and serum ferritin levels checked before resorting to a supplement.

THE CONVERSION OF FOOD TO FUEL

During physical activity the muscle cells convert energy obtained from the combustion of the fuels stored as glycogen in muscle, as fat in adipose tissue, and as circulating fuels (glucose and free fatty acids) into ATP (adenosine triphosphate – the fuel used for mechanical work). Additional energy can be obtained from the oral intake of nutrients, which adds to the circulating fuels in the blood.

Glycogen stored in the liver is broken down to glucose, which then enters the bloodstream from where it is extracted by the muscles and the brain. At rest this occurs at about 10g/hour and during exercise speeds up to about 60g/hour. Hypoglycaemia (low blood sugar levels) can develop in athletes who do not ingest adequate amounts of carbohydrate before and during prolonged exercise (considered to be 90 minutes or longer). Hypoglycaemia is an important cause of central nervous system fatigue (brain fatigue).

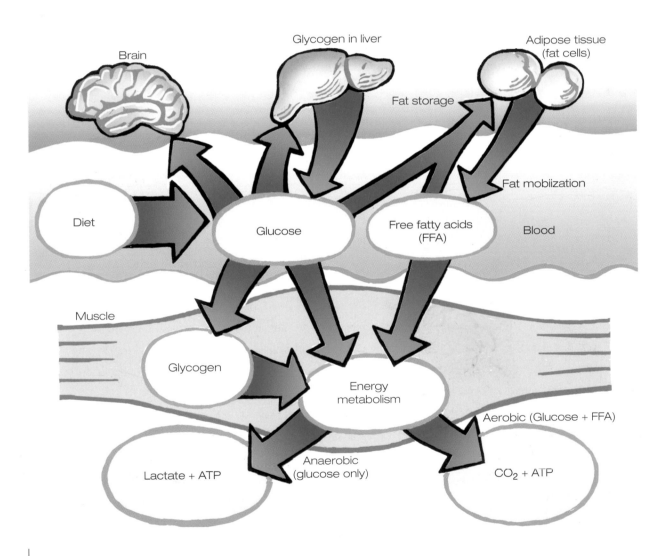

Above *From food to fuel.*

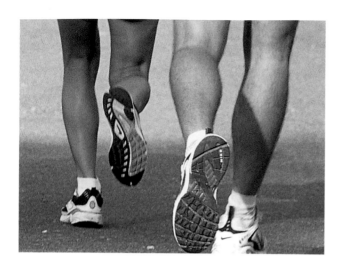

WHAT ABOUT LACTATE AND WHERE DOES IT FIT IN?

Lactate or lactic acid is often blamed for the burning feeling associated with fatigue and exhaustion during or just after maximal exercise and has also taken the blame for cramps, stitches, and for post-exercise muscle soreness. This is not the case and it is now widely accepted that the culprits are the production of hydrogen ions and the rise in muscle acidity. Supplements sold on the premise that lactate is a limiting factor in exercise therefore have no value (*see p103*).

Lactate, in fact, is a very important source of fuel. It is one of the products of glycolysis (the breakdown of glycogen). It is produced and used by the muscles. Its rate of production increases as the exercise intensity increases and as more carbohydrate is used as a fuel. Lactate from the muscle is either taken up by the liver and converted and stored as glycogen (via gluconeogenesis) or the lactate formed in the muscle can be shuttled to adjacent muscle fibres to be used as fuel to sustain exercise. It is thus not a useless byproduct of glycolysis, but is possibly an important metabolic fuel used by the muscles, especially during exercise (*see also Manipulating the Fuel Mix p30*).

Lactate is not the only factor responsible for fatigue. Studies have shown that fatigued runners can have varying blood lactate levels.

ENERGY SYSTEMS (HOW FUELS ARE USED)

ATP (adenosine triphosphate) is the energy that powers all cellular functions, including muscle contraction. There is only enough ATP in the muscle for a short burst (a few seconds) of muscular effort and it must be constantly replenished. (*See also p148.*) The body uses four different energy systems. They are:

- the (ATP-CP) phosphagen energy system. The ATP in the muscle and creatine phosphate collectively provide enough energy for 5–10 seconds of activity.
- the anaerobic glycolytic system involves metabolism of blood glucose and muscle glycogen in the absence of oxygen. This system is used predominantly in high-intensity exercise lasting from 30 seconds to 3 minutes. After one minute exercise becomes increasingly aerobic.
- the aerobic glycolytic system involves metabolism of carbohydrate in the presence of oxygen.
- the aerobic lipolytic system involves metabolism of fat in the presence of oxygen.

The muscles do not use one energy system exclusively, but a combination in which one will predominate, depending on the intensity and duration of exercise (*see graph opposite, top*). The work rate (power multiplied by duration) determines the total quantity of fuel used, while the intensity (power) determines the proportion of carbohydrate and fat oxidized. During moderately strenuous exercise that can be maintained for 90 minutes, less carbohydrate and more fat is used (*see graph opposite, bottom*). Regardless of the system used, carbohydrate is always a critical part of the fuel mix.

VO_2 max

One of the ways to measure fitness is by the volume of oxygen you can consume while exercising at your maximum capacity. This is expressed as VO_2 max – the maximum amount of oxygen in millilitres that you can use in one minute per kilogram of body weight.

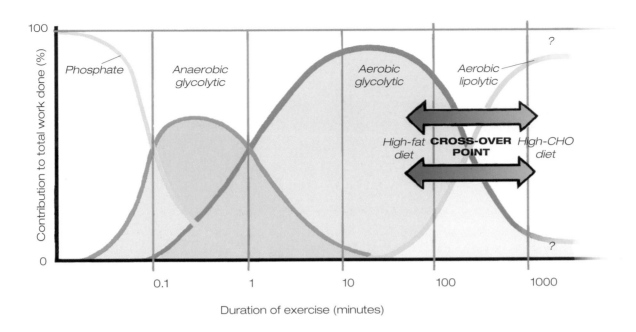

Above *Intensity and duration are the major determinants of the energy system used (see p30).*

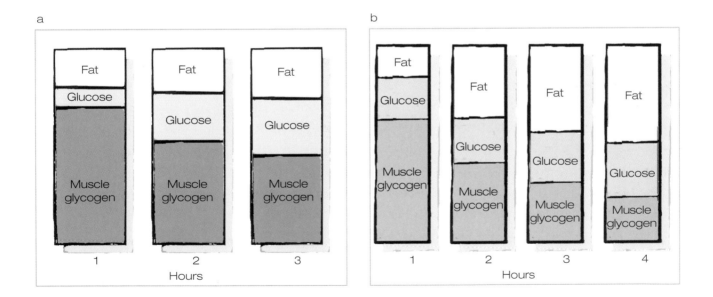

Above *Effect of duration and intensity of exercise on fuel oxidation (a) at 70% VO_2 max and (b) at 40% VO_2 max (adapted from Bosch et al, 1994).*

MANIPULATING THE FUEL MIX – HOW TO BECOME A BETTER FAT BURNER

Recent evidence shows that by manipulating training and diet you can alter the storage of carbohydrate and fat as well as their contribution to the fuel mix. Therefore, with an understanding of foods (the nutrients and fuel they provide) and the specific demands of particular sports, you can decrease one of the key factors causing fatigue and so optimize performance.

There are many anecdotal reports that athletes participating in different sporting events eat quite differently, instinctively selecting a diet to maximize their endurance. Many ultra-endurance athletes have been using high-fat diets. Documented dietary intakes in successful Antarctic crossings have been 57% fat, 34.6% carbohydrate and 8.4% protein of total energy intake. Mark Allen, six-times winner of the Hawaiian Ironman Triathlon (3.9km/2.4-mile swim, 180km/112-mile cycle, 42.2km/26-mile run) has said that he does not do well on a high-carbohydrate diet. 'It seemed like it was too low in protein and I personally needed a little more fat … so I didn't really tell people how I ate because it was so contrary to what was popular in the '80s.' Similarly, Paula Newby Fraser, eight-times winner of the women's Hawaiian Ironman Triathlon, admitted to not doing well on a traditional high-carbohydrate diet and has been quoted as saying: 'You can't train for the Ironman on pasta and salads.'

In support of these practices, sport scientists at the University of Cape Town have calculated that to complete the marathon (after having swum and cycled) in a time of 2hr 40min instead of 3hr 30min would require an additional 14.4kJ/min (60.5kcal/min). Because at this stage of the ultra-endurance event the energy from the body's own supplies of carbohydrate is depleted and exogenous carbohydrate (dietary carbohydrate provided by food/drink) cannot make up the difference, the only solution would be to increase the body's capacity to burn fat by 0.39g/min.

By manipulating your training and dietary regimes you can get your muscle to adapt to use more fat. Specific training causes several favourable changes in the energy systems you use. Firstly, your muscle is able to store more glycogen (double compared to an untrained athlete) and training also allows the liver to make more glycogen from lactate. Secondly, training also increases the capacity of the mitochondria to burn more fat (as a result of metabolic changes such as an increase in enzymes that are involved in fatty acid transportation and oxidation), as well as hormonal changes in plasma insulin and glucagon, which reduces fat storage.

Dietary manipulation is probably the most potent intervention that alters your capacity to burn more fat and so spare carbohydrate. The point at which fat and carbohydrate oxidation are equal (at a specific exercise intensity) is referred to as the cross-over (see graph p29). This can be shifted with dietary manipulation and training. Studies have shown that by increasing dietary fat to 70% of total energy intake (fat-loading) for about five days prior to prolonged exercise, the reliance on carbohydrate is decreased. This high-fat regime should be followed by a high-carbohydrate diet for one to three days. In this time the body is able to retool the mitochondria and adapt enzymes and hormones to burn fat, thereby slowing the rate of carbohydrate burning. For maximum benefit, the fat needs to be saturated (the less healthy animal fats) to create insulin resistance. Therefore, fat-loading can improve the mobilization of intra-muscular fat stores and limit glucose oxidation, which allows for prolonged exercise. (See fat-loading tips p166). However, there may be an increased perception of effort, so that this technique will not necessarily improve performance.

Many dietary supplements are marketed on the premise that they can change your ability to burn fat or carbohydrate. Caffeine, Medium-Chain Triglycerides (MCT), l-carnitine have all been promoted as so-called fat-burners. However, there is currently little evidence to support these effects and even in the case of caffeine, it loses its ability to mobilize fat in athletes who have carbohydrate-loaded (see p100).

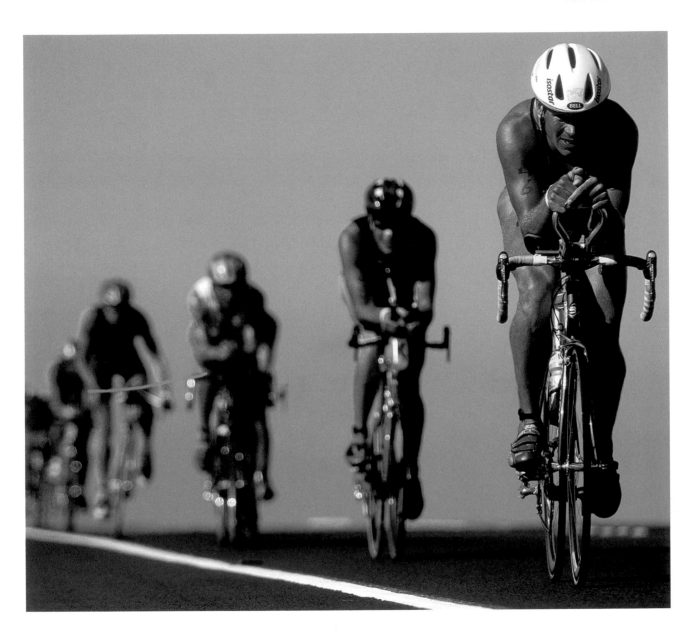

SUMMARY

New approaches are recognizing the different needs of each sport, sporting position, and sportsperson. These approaches take into account the different energy systems involved, as well as individual metabolic differences and adaptations to the different physiological demands. Furthermore, there are practical dietary constraints that need to be taken into consideration when planning diets for different events (24-hour swims, adventure racing, sailing). As a result, nutrition intervention is now becoming more specific with very different messages even for a sprinter, a middle-distance runner, a marathoner and an ultra-marathoner.

Above *Training and competing in ultra-endurance events needs specific dietary manipulation to meet the energy requirement, while taking practical considerations into account.*

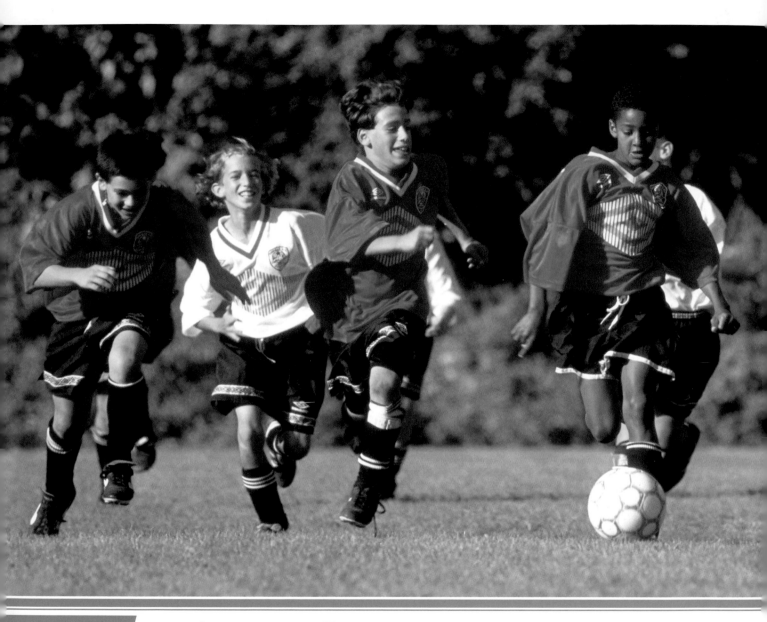

chapter 2

AGES AND STAGES

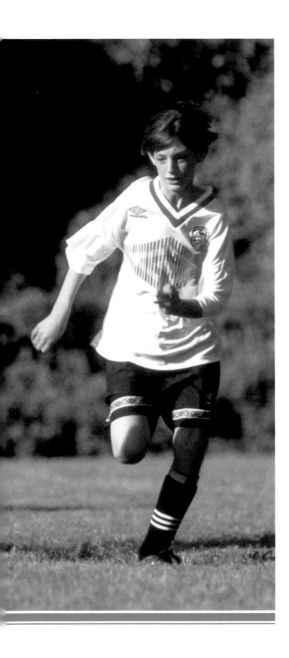

AGEING

The ageing process can be thought of as a continuum with a decrease in functional capacity, which is determined by genetics, lifestyle factors and chronic diseases. This process can be delayed by addressing lifestyle factors such as diet and exercise.

The nutritional requirements during different ages and stages of the life cycle will vary according to the specific demands on certain nutrients. The nutritional goals for sport change according to what happens to our bodies with age and these changes are highlighted in the sections below. Protein requirements are higher during childhood and adolescence for growth and maturation, whereas iron and calcium are important during pregnancy and lactation. For example, altered intake of fat may become a goal for an older exercising adult due to changes in fat deposition (body composition) during ageing.

CHILDREN AND YOUNG ATHLETES

GENERAL CONSIDERATIONS

In recent years, children's participation in high-level sports has become increasingly prevalent. If energy and nutrient intakes are not adequate to support the intense training, then growth and maturation may be delayed. In teenage girls menarche (onset of menstruation) may be delayed, which is a risk factor for menstrual dysfunction resulting in low peak bone density (see pp75–76). This is of great concern in aesthetic sports like gymnastics and ballet, where young athletes may severely restrict their energy intake to achieve lower body weights. In boys and girls total catch-up growth may be compromised if the delay in maturation is severe. In addition, immature bones are more susceptible to stress injuries.

The dietary needs and challenges of children and adolescents differ from those of adults. Fluid, for example, is a specific

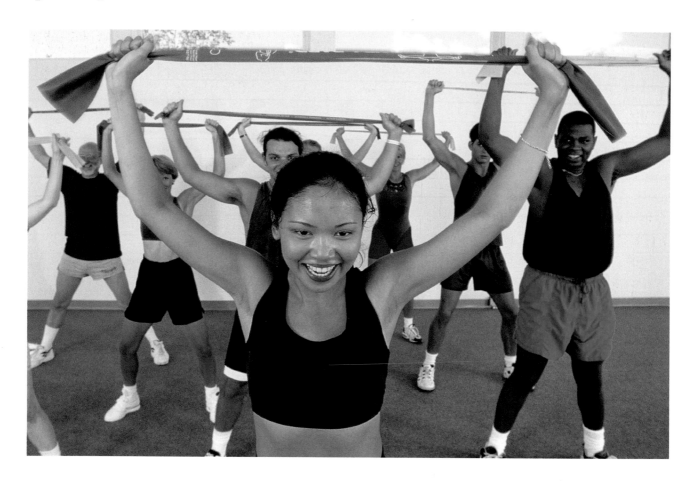

challenge for children because they do not tolerate extreme temperatures well and produce less sweat. Teenagers, especially those participating in competitive sport, are faced with additional challenges that include sexual maturation, change in body composition, rapid growth, coach, parent and peer pressure, scholastic achievement and social acceptance. In the pre-pubertal period the proportion of fat and muscle in girls and boys tends to be similar, with body fat being about 19 and 15% respectively. However, during puberty girls gain more body fat than boys (due to the laying down of energy reserves for pregnancy and lactation), whereas boys gain twice as much muscle mass. This causes

a lot of distress among many teenaged girls resulting in distorted body images, dieting and, in some cases, the development of eating disorders. Male teenagers on the other hand want to look more masculine and may use nutritional supplements to achieve this (see p98).

A multi-disciplinary approach involving parent, coach, young athlete and sports physician/dietitian with ongoing monitoring will help the early detection of any problems and establish lifelong healthy habits. Monitoring may involve measuring height, weight, skinfolds (see pp126, 127), pubertal stage, bone age, nutritional status, symptoms of eating disorders, and measures of body image.

Above *Children and teenagers require adequate energy and nutrients to support normal growth and development and the increased needs of training.*

Opposite top *The table shows the macronutrient requirements for exercising children and adolescents.*

NUTRITIONAL NEEDS

The diet of a healthy child should provide adequate energy and nutrients to support normal growth and the increased energy needs for training. It should always include a variety of foods. Population dietary goals and targets for children and adolescents can be used as guidelines for nutrient and energy intakes. These are known as the Recommended Dietary Allowances (RDAs) and Dietary Reference Intakes (DRIs). (*See p10 for values used in the United Kingdom.*) However, due to limited research on exercising children, specific requirements for sport still need to be established.

   * Energy The energy needs of healthy, growing children vary depending on their age, physical activity level and sex and it is therefore best to determine energy requirements on an individual basis using values such as the Estimated Energy Requirements (EER) and Physical Activity Levels (PAL) as broad guidelines (*see p10*). Note that adult values are not appropriate or suitable as they may underestimate the energy requirements of children who are less metabolically and mechanically efficient, therefore needing more energy for their body weight and height. They also need more energy for growth and maturation.

   ** Protein: Protein requirements are increased during childhood and adolescence to support growth and the additional demands of exercise and developing muscle mass. Protein intake should make up 15–20% of the total energy consumed and go up to 2g/kg body weight in male teenage athletes.

Children likely to be at risk for an inadequate protein intake include strict vegetarians or vegans, children with multiple food allergies or those who have limited food choices either because of fad diets or limited access to food, or who follow very high carbohydrate diets.

NUTRIENT	REQUIREMENT
ENERGY*	To support normal growth + energy needs of training
PROTEIN**	1.2–2g/kg
CARBOHYDRATE	>55% of total energy intake
FAT	30–35% of total energy intake

MICRONUTRIENTS

Provided the child meets the higher energy requirements and consumes a varied diet with nutrient-dense food choices, it is likely that they will meet their vitamin and mineral requirements and will thus not require vitamin and mineral supplementation.

   Minerals that are of great concern are iron, calcium and zinc. Iron is essential for haemoglobin formation and a deficiency can follow periods of rapid growth, which negatively impacts on sporting performance. In boys the gain in muscle mass is accompanied by an increase in blood volume and in girls iron is lost monthly due to menstruation. Iron-deficiency anaemia is a common problem in adolescent girls who are restricting their food intake because they think that they are fat. Calcium requirements for males and females increase substantially during adolescence to meet the demands of bone growth and to achieve a good bone mass. Zinc is also known to be essential for growth, but the retention of zinc increases during growth spurts, leading to more efficient use of dietary sources (*see table p24*).

   A child's diet should therefore be checked for these minerals, especially during periods of rapid growth (*see under Questions and Answers pp37, 38 and also p82*).

QUESTIONS PARENTS ASK

1. My 12-year-old daughter needs to lose weight for gymnastics. Can I cut her energy intake to 5000kJ (1200kcal) per day?

Severe and prolonged low-calorie diets are not recommended for young athletes since this may compromise the energy required for training, results in short stature and delays puberty, causes menstrual irregularities, increases the incidence of injuries and the risk of developing eating disorders. Therefore a diet of 5000kJ (1200kcal) may be too low, but an adequate calorie deficit can be achieved by simple lifestyle changes, such as better snack choices and less time spent watching TV. There is a very close correlation between the time spent watching TV and weight gain. Not only is this inactive time, but the advertising of fast foods and inappropriate snacks encourages poor food choices.

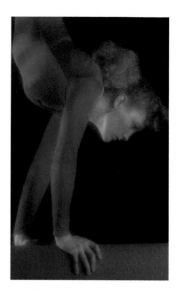

2. How much protein should young rugby players eat to build muscle?

Children and adolescents do require more protein than adults because of the extra protein required for growth. Protein is also required for gains in lean body mass and to compensate for protein used as a source of fuel in exercise and for muscle regeneration. However, there is a limit to the amount of protein that the muscle can use. It is also important to have sufficient carbohydrate together with the protein, because carbohydrate provides the necessary energy to fuel the work that the muscle must do to stimulate it to grow. It is therefore generally recommended that young rugby players consume 2g protein/kg body weight (for instance, a 60kg/132 lb player would need 120g protein per day).

Examples of low-fat foods that provide 10g protein per portion are listed on p22. See also p23 for practical tips.

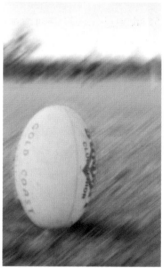

3. Will creatine help my son's soccer performance?

Creatine, an amino acid compound popularly taken as a supplement (*see p97*) is not recommended for children under the age of 18. In some situations and only in some individuals, creatine may enhance performance. However, it may have side effects and although a lot of these are anecdotal, no long-term studies have been done on adolescents. A concern with children taking creatine is that in a developing skeletal system, the increased force of the muscle (as a result of creatine supplementation) may lead to injury. Also, because water is transported into the muscle cells with creatine, large doses may be disadvantageous in the heat, especially in children who already are at risk for dehydration. Rather, they should stick to natural food sources of creatine – meat/fish/chicken/lean dried meat such as beef jerky. Some of these costly products may also contain ingredients that could be banned and at the end of the day the onus is on your son.

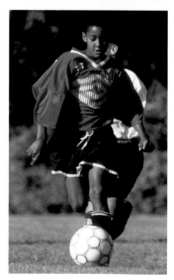

4. Should my talented child take a multivitamin or mineral supplement?

A daily vitamin and mineral supplement for well-fed, healthy, growing children is unnecessary, since their diets generally supply sufficient vitamins and minerals to meet their requirements. If parents wish to supplement their child or adolescent's diet with a multi-vitamin and mineral supplement, it is important to make sure that the supplement contains all or most of the vitamins and minerals according to the DRIs, or at least 50–150% of the DRIs. Some supplements do not contain enough iron, calcium and zinc or other minerals and therefore emphasis should be on achieving an adequate diet first. Megadoses of vitamins and minerals (doses greater than 10 x RDA) should be avoided as they may be toxic. The need for supplementation is, therefore, best addressed on an individual basis by a registered sports dietitian or medical doctor (*see p96*).

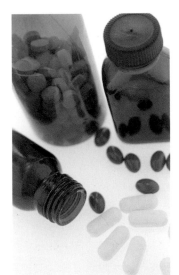

5. Are sports drinks necessary for young soccer players and how much should they drink?

Sports scientist Oded Bar-Or recommends the following broad guideline for children (1995): 'Drink periodically until not thirsty anymore, and then another few gulps.' Another few gulps would mean about 100–125ml (about ½ cup) beyond thirst for a child younger than 10 years and 200–250ml (¾–1 cup) beyond thirst for a child older than 10 years.

After training your child will still continue to lose fluid and so should continue drinking until he is urinating frequently.

Drinking is important to replace fluid losses and young athletes often begin training after school when they are already dehydrated. Fluids can also provide energy in the form of carbohydrate. Sports drinks provide both carbohydrate and fluid, but so does fruit juice (preferably diluted by 50%), diluted cordial, or even a carbohydrate powder when added to water. Although sports drinks may contain some other nutrients (for example, some electrolytes like sodium and potassium), snacks and food generally provide a more significant amount of these electrolytes. Some sports drinks may have added vitamin C, which is of course present in most fruit juices. So when it comes to choosing between any of the above drinks, choose what suits your pocket and a flavour that your child enjoys, since if he likes the taste he is likely to drink more.

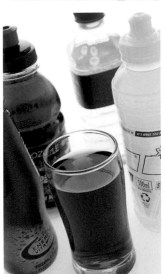

6. Is all this carbohydrate detrimental in terms of dental health?

Dental caries, or tooth decay, is the result of repeated acid attacks by bacteria on dental plaque. Sugars provide the energy for bacterial growth and the acids formed by the bacteria from the sugar substrate gradually erode the tooth enamel, causing decay. Two conditions accelerate the process: sticky carbohydrates that stick to tooth surfaces for a long time; and frequent exposure of tooth surfaces to sugar. In other words, the total

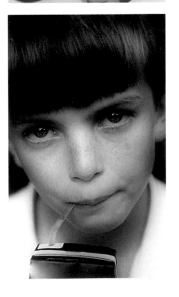

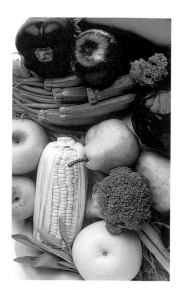

amount of sugar eaten is not as important in the formation of caries as the type of sugary food eaten, how often it is eaten and how long it sticks to the teeth. Sticky sweets are likely to be more harmful than a sports drink because, while providing the same amount of sugar, the drink is less likely to stick to the teeth for long. Eating five sticky sweets on five occasions during the day results in five exposures, while eating the five sweets at one time will reduce the total time of exposure. If eating or drinking sugary foods and beverages between meals, it is important to brush, floss and rinse the mouth afterwards.

Factors associated with dental caries:

- the physical form of the carbohydrate and the stickiness of the food
- the concentration of sugars in the foods consumed
- the length of time the teeth are exposed to acid
- the frequency of meals and snacks
- the proximity of eating to bedtime
- specific foods like citrus fruits and juices, carbonated and uncarbonated sugary drinks, acidic herbal teas, vinegar and vinegar products, sweets, acidic medications and supplements (for instance, vitamin C tablets and syrups).

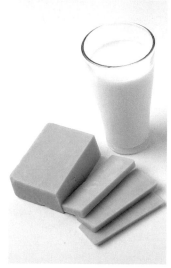

To prevent dental caries, encourage your child to:

- brush and floss teeth regularly (this is very important if your child wears braces)
- rinse the mouth frequently with water
- consume casein-containing food like milk and cheese
- chew sugar-free gum
- drink through a straw or squeeze-bottle, since this minimizes contact time with teeth
- have drinks chilled to reduce the erosive effects of acidic drinks
- always be adequately hydrated as this will promote saliva, which is an important buffer that prevents erosion.

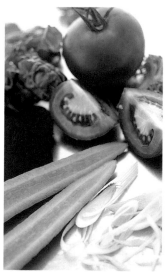

7. My son just refuses to eat fruit and vegetables. Can he simply replace this with a vitamin and mineral supplement?

The best strategy to obtain adequate nutrients in a form that is well absorbed by the body is to eat a variety of food. Of course, fruit and vegetables are especially rich in many vitamins, minerals and other phyto-nutrients. However, 91% of children aged 6–11 years do not consume the recommended minimum of five servings of fruit and vegetables per day. Most children average 2½ servings a day, making it difficult to achieve adequate intakes of many vitamins. If your child has a particular aversion to fruit or vegetables, try some of the following tips before buying a supplement:

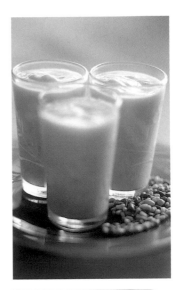

- Add vegetables to stews, soups (even puréed), casseroles, stir-fries, and to meat or chicken kebabs.
- Encourage fruit-based desserts (apple sauce, baked apple, fruit kebabs).
- Make fruit salad (often a child is too lazy to cut up the fruit).
- Dried fruit is a concentrated source of many nutrients.
- Fruit and vegetable juices or smoothies should take preference over colddrinks. 125ml (½ cup) fruit juice counts as a fruit serving.

8. Should my child only eat carbohydrate foods that are rich in fibre?

Children older than two years should aim for a daily fibre intake equal to their age plus 5g. Good sources of fibre include high-fibre cereals, wholegrain breads and crackers, oats porridge, legumes, fruit and vegetables. Avoid excessive fibre intake, which may reduce consumption of much-needed energy and nutrients, especially in active children. First ensure that your child achieves the basic fibre requirement beyond which you can be more flexible and include carbohydrate foods with less fibre.

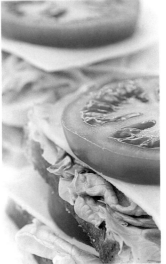

9. My child is constantly tired. Can this be related to his diet?

Yes, although there are other factors, like overtraining and lack of adequate sleep. Check on your child's overall energy, carbohydrate and protein intake, as well as certain vitamins (for instance, the B-vitamins) and minerals. Lack of dietary iron, for example, may cause fatigue. Rich sources of iron include meat, chicken, beef jerky, liver, spinach and some dried fruits. Post-training nutrition is also a factor. After exercise, there is a window period of 1–2 hours when the muscles have an accelerated ability to replace carbohydrate stores. Ensure that your child has something to eat after training, particularly if he spends time travelling home from training: aß sandwich with a filling of cheese, fruit-flavoured yoghurt, a carbohydrate drink, fruit juice, a few crackers, a raisin bun, or a cereal/sports bar. Provided the snack supplies sufficient carbohydrate (about 50g – see p17) you can include some protein. Protein is especially important if there has been any muscle damage.

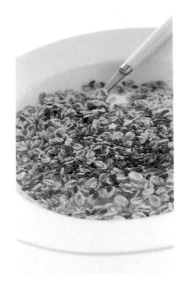

10. When my son goes away on cricket tour, how can I ensure that he eats properly?

If your child does not enjoy trying new foods or you are concerned about the food on tour, it is always a good idea to pack a supply of familiar foods to take with. Fresh and dried fruit, crackers, pretzels, muesli and breakfast bars, dry cereal (in serve-size packets), skim-milk powder, a tin of low-fat liquid meal replacement powder, fruit juices, instant oats or quick-cooking noodles (if a kettle is available), and carbohydrate powders are suitable options.

PREGNANCY AND LACTATION

GENERAL CONSIDERATIONS: PREGNANCY POINTERS

If you are planning to become pregnant and have irregular or absent periods, you may have to reduce your training intensity and/or increase your body fat a little. This will improve your chances of conception and help ensure an optimal birth weight for your baby. Supplementation with folate will help prevent neural-tube defects. Poor weight gain during pregnancy also increases the risk of a low birth weight baby. A low body fat percentage is associated with lower sex hormones.

The factors that determine your training and nutrition programme in pregnancy are your pre-pregnancy fitness, type of sport, training demands, comfort, adequate weight gain, morning sickness, and the presence of other risk factors.

NUTRITIONAL NEEDS

- Energy intake should be adequate to meet the extra energy needs not only of pregnancy, but also of the exercise performed. Note that in pregnancy, activity levels may be reduced and so the additional energy requirements for exercise may be minimal.

- Extra calories are not required until the second and third trimesters of pregnancy when an additional 1260kJ (300kcal) are recommended. Adding in an extra 1–2 cups of low-fat milk, yoghurt or low-fat cheese plus an extra portion of protein of choice can help achieve increased requirements for protein, calcium and energy. Some women may need more than this depending on their size, activity level and nutritional status. Appropriate weight gain during the pregnancy indicates whether sufficient calories are being provided.

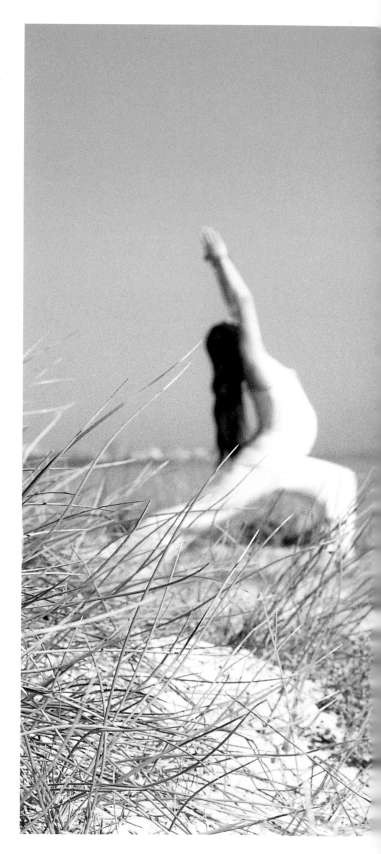

Right *Dietary requirements for specific nutrients increase during pregnancy to meet the needs of the developing foetus, as well as those of the exercising mother.*

■ Do not attempt to restrict your intake or go on a diet during pregnancy.

■ There is an increased need for most vitamins and minerals in pregnancy, and the most important ones include calcium, iron, zinc, folic acid, vitamin C, vitamin D and B vitamins. If you continue to exercise regularly throughout your pregnancy, it is important to monitor your iron status.

■ Eat plenty of folate-rich foods (for example, wholegrain cereals, eggs, legumes), fruit and vegetables and take a supplement containing 360–800µg of folic acid in the pre-conception period and in the first trimester.

■ Avoid vitamin A supplements or eating excessive amounts of liver. Excessive vitamin A may be toxic to the foetus.

■ Your diet should contain enough essential fatty acids to support the growth and development of your baby's brain and central nervous system. Good sources of essential fatty acids include nuts, seeds, vegetable oils, oily fish and fish oils.

■ Drink plenty of fluids before, during and after exercise to reduce the risk of thermal stress. Ensure that your body temperature does not exceed 38°C (100.4°F). Monitor your heartbeat and ensure that it does not exceed 140 beats per minute. Exercise in well-ventilated surroundings and allow extra time for cooling down.

■ It is recommended that women avoid alcohol during their pregnancy, especially during the first 12 weeks and during breastfeeding. However, the odd glass of wine or beer after the first 12 weeks is not considered by some to be a risk – as long as it is limited to 1 unit a day or less (*see alcohol, p69*).

■ Lactation: You need to eat small, frequent snacks that are energy and nutrient dense (fruit yoghurt, dried fruit, smoothies, energy and breakfast bars, cheese and crackers, pita wedges with hummus) throughout the day to get the extra energy needed for breastfeeding and exercise. Note that milk production may be reduced on low energy intakes or if exercising excessively, so rapid weight loss and low-energy diets are not advised. Ensure adequate

fluid intakes during breast-feeding. Exercise alters the taste of breast milk because of the lactic acid build-up in the milk. Plan to breast-feed before exercise or express and store breast milk for post-exercise feeds.

■ Exercise tips: continue your regular training programme throughout pregnancy, provided you feel well. Gradually reduce the training intensity and volume as pregnancy progresses. Aim to maintain rather than increase your fitness. Avoid any activity that places excessive pressure, stress or movement on any joint because the ligaments are more lax during pregnancy. Excessive exercise together with inadequate energy intake can lead to sub-optimal weight gain and poor foetal growth. Therefore, exercise should be moderate. Do not exercise if you feel fatigued, nauseous or dizzy.

MASTER ATHLETES

GENERAL CONSIDERATIONS

With the knowledge that exercise delays the ageing process and improves health, the number of older individuals partici-pating in regular exercise is on the increase. The ageing process is accompanied by many physiological changes that affect nutritional needs (*see table opposite*). In addition there are other factors to consider in an older person, such as chronic degener-ative diseases (for example, coronary heart disease, hypertension, dia-betes mellitus), decreased sensitivity to taste and smell, decreased appetite, and increased use of medica-tion, which may affect nutrient absorption. Fluid needs are increased due to a loss of thirst sensitivity and a delay in the sweat response. Thus older athletes need to be more aware of their fluid requirements during exercise.

AGE-RELATED CHANGES THAT MAY INFLUENCE NUTRIENT REQUIREMENTS IN OLDER ATHLETES

Reduced muscle mass, aerobic capacity, glycogen stores, bone density, calcium bioavailability, vitamin D syn-thesis, immune function, metabolic use of pyridoxine (B_6), gastric acid, hepatic uptake of retinol, thirst perception, kidney function.

Increased oxidative stress (*see p89*), homocysteine levels (*see glossary*).

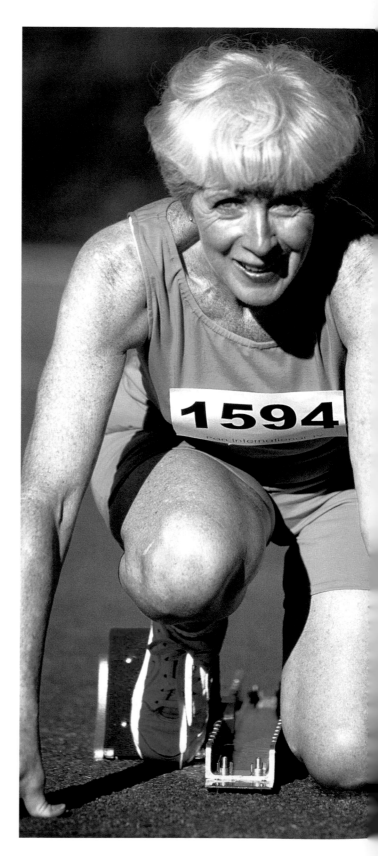

Right *Fluid requirements are increased in older athletes due to a loss of thirst sensitivity and a delay in the sweat response.*

NUTRITIONAL NEEDS

Recommendations for nutrition in ageing athletes should focus on both the nutritional requirements of the ageing process and the nutrient needs for exercising.

An older athlete has a lower daily energy requirement due to decreases in muscle mass, aerobic capacity and the decreased capacity to store muscle glycogen (due to reduced muscle mass). For protein, carbohydrate and fat, requirements are given as ranges because the specific amount will vary depending on the individual's health status and goals. For example, older athletes with raised blood cholesterol levels may need to keep their fat intake to the lower end of the range, whereas someone needing to lose weight may respond to a higher protein diet.

There is an increased need for calcium and vitamin D to reduce the rate at which bone density is lost. Vitamins B_6 and E and zinc are important for immune function. The recommendations given for the B vitamins folate, pyridoxine and B_{12} are based on their ability to lower homocysteine levels, a known risk factor for the development of coronary heart disease. Note, however, that there are upper limits of safety and that excessive dosages are unsafe. Zinc and iron intakes are often low in older people, especially if they are vegetarian. Master athletes should therefore always aim to achieve the RDAs/DRVs for these nutrients (*see pp82, 89*). Calcium requirements for men and women increase from 1000 to 1200mg/day over the age of 51 years with an upper limit of safety of 2500mg/day. DRVs in the United Kingdom differ (*see p10*). Dietary sources of vitamin C will enhance the absorption of all of these minerals.

NUTRIENT	DAILY REQUIREMENT
MACRONUTRIENTS	
Energy	Basal requirements decrease, although extra is needed to cover training
Protein	1.2–1.7g per kg body weight
Carbohydrate	50–60%
Fat	20–30%
MICRONUTRIENTS	
Vitamin B_6	2mg
Vitamin B_{12}	3.6µg
Folate	400µg
Vitamin D	51–70 years: 10µg; >70years >15µg/day
Calcium	1200mg (>65 years)

Above *Some suggested intakes for master athletes, taking physical activity into account.*
Below *Vitamin C-rich foods, like citrus, enhance the absorption of iron, calcium and zinc.*

 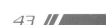

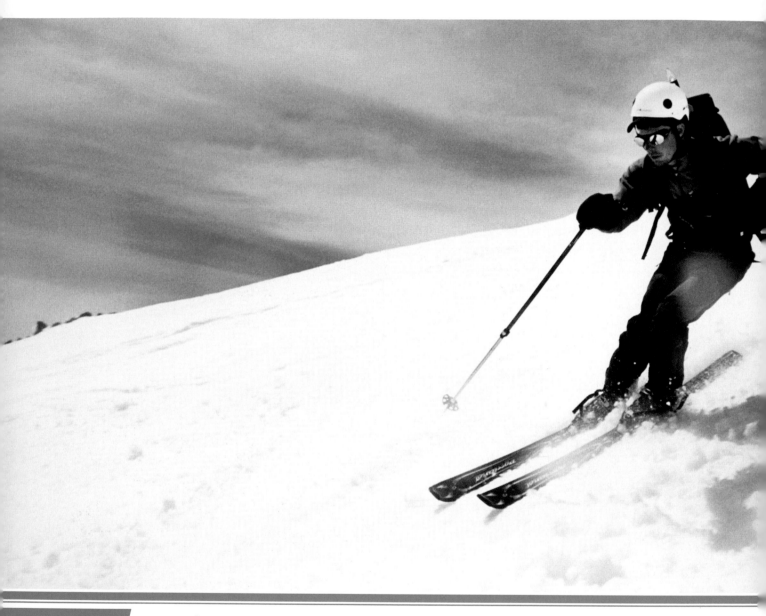

chapter 3

MAKING A PLAN

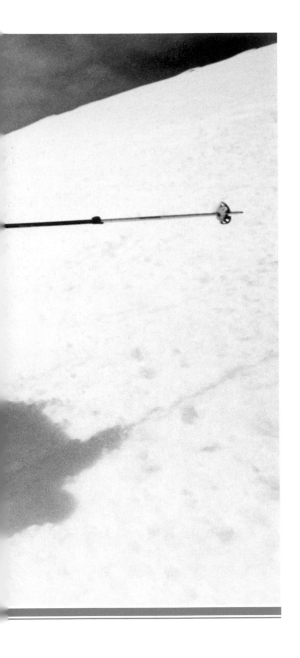

THE SCIENCE AND ART OF EATING

A winning diet involves both the science and the art of eating. The science is the knowledge of what you should be eating for your sport, and the art is putting this knowledge into practice. Strategies that can meet several nutrition goals simultaneously are required, as all of these separate issues need to be integrated to optimize your overall sports performance. These issues include poor nutrition knowledge; dietary extremism; lack of practical skills in choosing or preparing meals; and limited access to food due to financial constraints, busy lifestyles or frequent travel.

This chapter provides you with all the tools needed to put your Nutrition Game Plan into action!

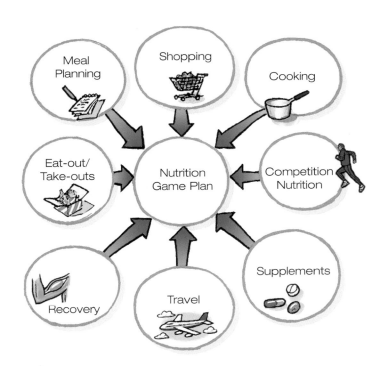

Above *Typical challenges and lifestyle factors that affect nutrition goals and therefore performance.*

MEAL PLANNING

You need a basic understanding of your carbohydrate, protein and fat requirements to plan your meals.

The example below shows the average macronutrient requirements of an 80kg (176 lb) athlete training two hours per day and how these nutrient goals can be translated into a practical daily meal plan.

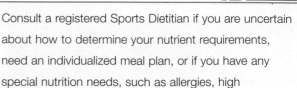

Tip

Consult a registered Sports Dietitian if you are uncertain about how to determine your nutrient requirements, need an individualized meal plan, or if you have any special nutrition needs, such as allergies, high cholesterol levels or need a vegetarian diet, for instance.

MACRONUTRIENT	CARBOHYDRATE	PROTEIN	FAT
DAILY REQUIREMENTS PER KG OF BODY WEIGHT PER DAY	5–7g/kg	1–2.2g/kg	1–1.5g/kg (20–30% of total daily energy intake)
RECOMMENDED DAILY INTAKE	500g (6g/kg body weight)	100g (130g minus 30g to account for the 30g protein contained in some of the carbohydrate-rich foods)	26g (80g ÷ 3, since fat is found in many of the protein- and carbohydrate-rich foods and snacks, your 'added' fat intake should be limited to ⅓ of your total daily fat allowance)
FOOD SOURCES	50g carbohydrate servings to choose from: 500ml (2 cups) porridge 3 fruit 3 slices bread 250ml (1 cup) fruit yoghurt 250ml (1 cup) pasta 40ml (3½tbsp) raisins 2 sports bars 750ml (1½pt) sports drink	10g protein servings. to choose from: 40g (1⅓ oz) chicken 300ml (1¼ cup) low-fat milk 2 eggs 50g (1.7 oz) tuna 30g (1 oz) low-fat hard cheese	5g fat servings to choose from: 5ml (1tsp) soft margarine 12.5ml (1tbsp) low-fat mayonnaise ¼ avocado pear 5ml (1tsp) olive oil

Above *A table showing examples of food from which to calculate a meal plan that meets your requirements.*

Total daily energy intake = 13,600kJ (3240kcal)

This should be split into several meals and snacks.

Your meal-planning checklist:

√ variety – include new foods, new recipes, and variety within each group

√ mix and match foods at all your meals, using the plate model on p23 as your template

√ do not exclude any food group for any reason

√ include adequate fluid.

Adjust your carbohydrate intake according to your training:

■ for 1 hour training per day: reduce carbohydrate intake to 5g/kg of body weight

■ for more than 2 hours training per day: increase carbohydrate intake to 7–8g/kg of body weight

■ for no training (off-season or when injured) reduce carbohydrate intake further and reduce protein and fat intakes to the low end of the ranges in the table above.

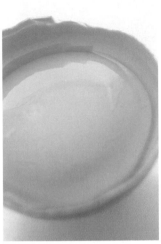
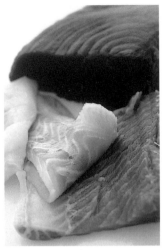
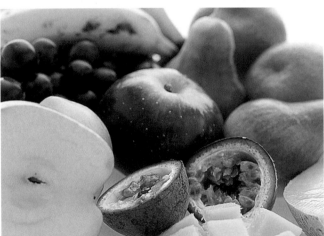
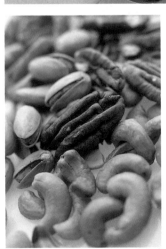

BREAKFAST

500ml (2 cups) porridge + 300ml (1¼ cup) low-fat milk + 1 fruit

MID-MORNING

2 slices bread + 5ml (1tsp) margarine + 30g (1 oz) low-fat hard cheese + tomato slices + 1 fruit

LUNCH

4 slices bread + 25ml (2tbsp) low-fat mayonnaise + 1 boiled egg + 50g (1.7 oz) tuna + ¼ avocado pear + salad + 1 fruit

MID-AFTERNOON

250ml (1 cup) low-fat fruit yoghurt + 40ml (3½tbsp) raisins

SUPPER

240g (8 oz) chicken (no skin) + 500ml (2 cups) pasta + 10ml (2tsp) olive oil + vegetables of choice

SNACKS AND DRINKS TO BE EATEN BEFORE/DURING/AFTER TRAINING

2 sports bars + 750ml (1½pt) sports drink

(For food alternatives see 50g carbohydrate list p17.)

Above right *Sample one-day meal plan for an 80kg (176 lb) athlete providing 13,600kJ (3240kcal).*

FREEZER LIST

Skinless chicken, crumbed chicken breasts and chicken sausage

Lean beef, ostrich, lamb or pork fillets, cubes, strips or mince

Frozen vegetables and stir-fry mixes

Bread, rolls, pita breads, raisin buns/bread

Pizza bases

Muffins, crumpets, pancakes

Grated low-fat cheese (for instance, Mozzarella)

Oven-baked chips

FRIDGE LIST

Fresh fruit, vegetables and juices

Low-fat cheese

Low-fat milk and yoghurt

Buttermilk

Low-fat custard

Eggs

Margarine, butter, low-fat mayonnaise

Lean cold-meat cuts and chicken and turkey

SNACK CUPBOARD

Cereal bars, sports bars, muesli bars

Instant oats sachets, cereals

Quick noodles

Dried fruit

Low-fat crackers

Peanut butter, cheese spread, chocolate spread, honey, jam, syrup

Processed cheese wedges or spreads – low fat

Tins of baked beans

Pretzels

Unbuttered popcorn

Plain sweet biscuits

FOOD CUPBOARD/PANTRY

Pasta, quick-cooking noodles, rice, couscous, polenta, samp

Oats, mealiemeal (maize flour), breakfast cereals

Crumpet/pancake mixes

Canned and dried legumes (kidney beans, baked beans, lentils, chickpeas)

Cream-style sweet corn

Canned tomato and tomato/onion mixes

Canned non-cream tomato and vegetable soups

Canned fruit

Tinned fish (tuna, pilchards, sardines)

Long-life milk

Long-life custard or custard powder

Bottled pasta sauces (tomato, for instance)

Soy sauce

Vinegar

Dried herbs and spices

Sugar

Flour

Cocoa and other milkshake powders

Jams, honey, syrup, peanut butter, yeast (vegetable) extract and fish paste

Oil cooking sprays

Skim milk powder

Jelly

Cordials: powder or syrup form

Sports drinks

Oil

Above *Create varied and interesting quick-to-prepare meals using these foods in different combinations to avoid menu fatigue.*

SHOPPING

Plan a week's menu and make a shopping list. Include different carbohydrates (rice, potato, pasta) and proteins (meat, chicken, fish and legumes), vegetables and fruit for variety. Stock basic items and top up with fresh produce once or twice a week. Long-life products are useful if you live in a boarding house or residence.

FOOD LABELS – READ BETWEEN THE LINES

- Ingredients on food packages are listed in descending order of weight. If fat (lard, butter, vegetable oil, hydrogenated/palm kernel oil, cream, coconut milk) is high on the list, the product is probably high in fat.
- Claims should be backed up. For instance, if 'low fat', values of fat should be given.
- When comparing products check that the values are in the same units and relate this to the amount you eat.
- The energy content of food may be expressed as calories (kcal) or kilojoules (kJ). Multiply kcal by 4.2 for kJ.
- Cholesterol-free does not mean fat-free. It is only found in animal products.
- Health products may be free from preservatives and additives, but can still be high in fat.
- Check the 'best before' or 'use by' dates.

STRETCHING YOUR FOOD BUDGET

Meet your sports nutrition goals without chewing through your budget.

- Prepare your own food.
- Add beans and lentils to mince to 'stretch' the protein.
- Instead of carbonated beverages buy cordials, powders, and concentrated juices or sports drinks.
- Instead of chocolates and sweets, buy fruit, fruit rolls, canned fruit, jelly, low-fat flavoured yoghurt, drinking yoghurt, and low-fat custard.
- Instead of pies and hot potato chips, buy or make sandwiches or rolls or baked potatoes with low-fat fillings.

- A cost-effective way to boost your protein and carbohydrate intake is to add skim milk powder to milk, milk drinks, porridge, cereals and mashed potatoes.

COOKING AND FOOD PREPARATION

REDUCE THE FAT IN FOOD PREPARATION

- Grill, bake on a rack or in foil, barbecue, microwave, steam, or 'dry fry' with a nonstick frying pan (with a smear of oil or a spray) to prevent food from sticking.
- Limit the amount of oil to 1–2 teaspoons per person when preparing a meal.
- Lemon juice, low-fat yoghurt, wine or stock can be used to baste or marinade food to prevent it from drying out.
- Modify recipes to use reduced-fat ingredients: plain yoghurt or reduced-fat cream instead of cream, and skim or low-fat milk instead of full-cream milk, etc.
- Replace roast and fried food with dry-baked items.
- Herbs, spices, lemon juice or crumbs can be used to flavour vegetables instead of margarine, oil or butter.

TO INCREASE THE NUTRIENT-DENSE CARBOHYDRATE CONTENT

- Add lentils to white or brown rice.
- Include vegetables, salads and fruit at every meal.
- Add beans or lentils to soups and stews.
- Fresh or stewed fruit can be enjoyed as a dessert.
- Leftover rice and pasta can be frozen – to reheat, microwave or pour boiling water over it and drain, or use quick-cooking noodles or couscous.

EAT-OUTS AND TAKE-OUTS

Eating out can give you a much-needed break. By making careful choices with clever combinations, and keeping to your recommended portion sizes, your dietary goals can still be met. When eating out, don't eat entirely out of character; decide what your nutrition goals are and stick to them.

RESTAURANT	RECOMMENDED	
ITALIAN	Italian breads without added butter, insalata (green salad) or caprese (tomato and Mozzarella salad); minestrone (add little Parmesan); marinated calamari; pasta with vegetable or tomato-based sauce, or a lean meat (bolognaise), chicken or a non-creamy seafood sauce; thick-based pizza with half the amount of cheese and vegetable or fruit toppings with the option of lean ham/chicken/tuna. For dessert, order fat-free sorbet or fresh fruit, or cappuccino (with foam).	
CHINESE, THAI, MALAYSIAN	Steamed rice or noodles, topped with stir-fried meat, vegetables or tofu; chicken or a prawn steamed meal. Request that stir-fries be cooked only with a little oil. Clear broth soups.	
INDIAN	Steamed rice – use as a base for the meal; lentils; chickpeas; vegetable, chicken or fish curry. Indian breads (pulkas, naan – no butter). Mulligatawny soup or a lentil soup. For dessert, opt for khur, a sweetened rice pudding or a lassi (yoghurt drink).	
MEXICAN	Order individual items from the menu rather than large, set main courses. Choose rice, beans, tortillas or a fajita. Good fillings include a combination of salsa, rice salad and char-grilled beef or chicken strips or beans. Gazpacho or black bean soup. Choose fruit for dessert.	
GREEK	Dolmades, grilled calamari (without a butter sauce, and not deep fried), lean souvlaki (lamb marinated in garlic, lemon juice and olive oil), tzaziki (yoghurt, garlic, cucumber), hummus (chick peas and sesame paste) with pita bread. Fish baked in a tomato sauce. Plenty of rice and orzo (rice pasta).	
JAPANESE	Control your fat intake by ordering foods that are yaki (broiled or grilled), nimono (simmered), or variations thereof. For example, beef teriyaki and chicken yakitori. Sashimi (raw fish) and sushi (vinegared rice prepared with seaweed, raw fish and/or vegetables). Cesium with shredded wasabi (strong horseradish sauce), tofu dishes and miso (fermented soybean) soup are good options.	
AFRICAN	Ostrich and venison, lean bredies (stews) or curries, lean mince or fish bobotie (casserole) and smoorsnoek (braised fish). Samp (crushed maize) and beans, pap (maize porridge). Desserts include sago pudding, crustless milk tart (custard tart), bread-and-butter pudding and pancakes with cinnamon, sugar or fruit.	
FAST FOODS	Salad or chicken burger or steak sandwich with chutney or tomato, barbecue or monkey gland sauce. Chicken kebab or char-grilled chicken with rolls or pita bread or rice. Baked potato topped with low-fat cheese or lean meat, chicken and mushrooms. Sandwiches, wraps, subs or rolls with lean meat, chicken, cottage cheese or fish with lots of salads. Lean meat or vegetable curry with rice. Corn salad or three-bean salad.	

AVOID

Pasta with a creamy sauce (Alfredo or carbonara); lots of cheese, lasagne and cannelloni as these can be very high in fat; fatty meat; pizza with lots of cheese and fatty meat toppings; heavily smoked and salted meats (salami and pepperoni) and cheeses served with antipasto.

(Watch the oil!) Battered or deep-fried foods (crispy); fried rice; spring rolls and deep-fried finger foods; anything cooked in coconut cream or milk; duck.

Fried or battered foods (or dishes prepared with ghee or coconut milk); samoosas; fried breads; meat curries and fried vegetables. Thick cheese puddings and honeyed pastries.

Cheese; sour cream; fatty meat; corn chips; nachos.

Fatty meats; moussaka and pastitsio. Limit the use of olive oil. Casseroles made with plenty of eggs and cheese. Baklava.

Tempura, agemono and katsu refer to foods that are breaded and fried.

Pies and samoosas (pastries), boerewors (fried sausage) and ribs, fritters and koeksisters (tye of syrup doughnut).

Fried fish and chips. Crumbed and fried chicken. Toasted sandwiches with butter on both sides.

Practical Tips

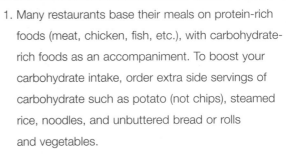

1. Many restaurants base their meals on protein-rich foods (meat, chicken, fish, etc.), with carbohydrate-rich foods as an accompaniment. To boost your carbohydrate intake, order extra side servings of carbohydrate such as potato (not chips), steamed rice, noodles, and unbuttered bread or rolls and vegetables.

2. To limit your fat intake avoid battered, fried, deep-fried, sautéed, creamy, creamed and crumbed foods. Rather choose dishes that are steamed, grilled, flame-grilled, stir-fried, baked or poached. Remind waitrons that NO fat means NO oil, margarine, butter or cream.

3. Don't be misled by the word 'healthy' – this does not necessarily mean low in fat. For example, salads may seem 'healthy', but may be high in fat if they contain avocado, cheese, seeds and croutons, which are high in fat. Dressings should be ordered on the side, so that you can control the amount you add to your food, or use balsamic vinegar with a dash of olive oil.

4. Avoid creamy sauces, gravies, dressings, butter, creamy foods and foods with lots of cheese (e.g. vegetarian). Ask for sauces to be served separately. Combination dishes such as baked pastas, casseroles and moussaka are often made with high-fat sauces, so rather order plain, separate food items, such as grilled fish or meat, baked potato and steamed rice and vegetables. Mint sauce, jelly, mustard, horseradish and apple sauce can be enjoyed with different meats.

5. For dessert, order fruit salad with a fruit sorbet or a meringue/pavlova with frozen yoghurt, fruit mousse, plain sponge or a cappuccino.

COMPETITION NUTRITION

There are many factors that may affect nutritional requirements for competitive events and depending on the type of event, dietary strategies would need to be individually tailored. Team-based, multiday events; ultra-endurance races; weight-category sports; and track and field events all require a different dietary strategy before, during and after the competition. These strategies are dictated by the physiological demands of the sport as well as practical considerations specific to the sport. Chapters 8 to 13 cover the specific dietary requirements of the different sports in detail. There are, however, some general guidelines which can be applied to all sports and situations.

PRE-COMPETITION NUTRITION [WEEK BEFORE]

PRINCIPLES

In the week leading up to an event, all that should be required is the fine-tuning of your already well-planned training and eating regime. You would have tried and tested different approaches as well as foods and sports drinks to determine what works best for you to avoid trying anything new at this stage. You should also be close to your competition weight.

You may need to maximize your fuel stores, especially if you are competing in prolonged events. Generally, if your event lasts longer than 90 minutes, you may need to consider carbohydrate-loading techniques (*see p165*) and if your event is less than 90 minutes, your already high-carbohydrate training diet coupled with adequate rest is all you need to ensure adequate fuel stores.

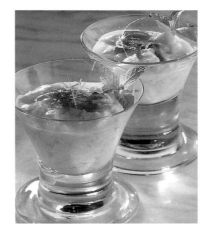
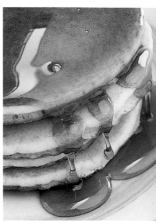

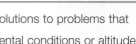
Tips

- Think ahead and consider solutions to problems that may arise through environmental conditions or altitude for example, so that you can plan accordingly.
- If extra carbohydrate is needed over and above your daily intake, focus on more concentrated carbohydrate foods such as sports drinks, sugar, etc.
- Resist the temptation to try something new. Don't be influenced by strategies used by competitors – what works for them may not work for you. Remember each sport and situation is unique – if you are a sprinter or a jockey, you don't need to carbo-load.
- You may need to select and focus on the most important events during the year to avoid the consequences of overtraining, which could be compounded by chronic extreme dietary strategies.
- Schedule and modify training sessions, which could damage muscle fibres, for a few days before the competition to allow more time for recovery.
- Remain well hydrated at all times (*see pp58–69*).
- Travel, eating in foreign destinations, social functions and event management may challenge your typical training regime and therefore affect your pre-event nutrition (*see Travel Tips p57*).

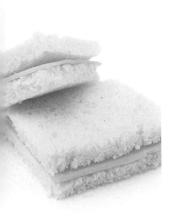
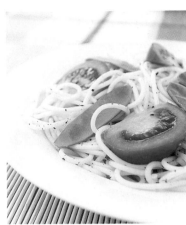

PRE-COMPETITION NUTRITION (MEAL BEFORE)

PRINCIPLES

Use this opportunity to top up your liver glycogen stores (especially after an overnight fast) and also to hydrate. Choose foods and drinks that do not cause any gastro-intestinal discomfort and that will stave off hunger pangs. This meal should also give you the psychological edge and boost your confidence before competing.

EXAMPLES OF PRE-COMPETITION MAIN MEALS:

- spaghetti or other noodles with a little lean mince and/or vegetable or tomato-based topping (no cream)
- chicken à la king and rice served with peas and carrots
- grilled chicken breast with mashed potato, sweet potato or stir-fried rice
- baked potato with tuna, chicken or vegetable-based topping.

Extra bread, fruit, fruit salad and low-fat yoghurt or low-fat desserts can be included with this meal plus sports drinks. You will need to consume a lighter top-up snack 1–2 hours before the event.

EXAMPLES OF PRE-COMPETITION TOP-UP SNACKS:

- sandwiches with either low-fat cheese, ham, chicken, boiled egg, tuna, jam or peanut butter
- muffins or pancakes or crumpets with honey or syrup or sugar and cinnamon
- fresh fruit and low-fat yoghurt
- fruit smoothies
- sports bars or cereal/breakfast bars and sports drinks
- low-fibre breakfast cereal and low-fat milk or yoghurt
- low-fat rice pudding.

If you lack appetite or if you cannot tolerate solid food, a liquid meal replacement is an option.

Choose foods high in carbohydrate and low in fat, also low in fibre and bulk to avoid diarrhoea.

You should always begin your event well hydrated, especially in events when the weather is hot and humid. Immediately before an endurance event drink about 250–500ml (½–1pt) of a carbohydrate-electrolyte sports drink as this primes the stomach and assists with fluid emptying and meets both fluid and carbohydrate needs. Leave time for a toilet stop before the start. In shorter events water may be sufficient before the event (*see tips on hydration p64*).

If you are unable to eat prior to an endurance event, it is critical to consume 50–60g carbohydrates per hour during the event to avoid hypoglycaemia.

Tips

- Timing of the meal and the quantity of food eaten will vary from individual to individual. The key is to find out what works for you and stick to it.
- If a large meal is to be consumed, allow 3–4 hours before the event for digestion.

Above *Ideas for light pre-competition meals.*

Myth or Truth? Should carbohydrates, especially high GI carbohydrates (*see p17*), be avoided within one hour of an event?

Previously, it was believed that a high GI carbohydrate intake prior to an event causes blood insulin levels to peak with a subsequent drop in blood sugar levels resulting in hypoglycaemia. Recent studies show that, although insulin levels do increase after consuming high GI foods (*see pp17, 85*) and that blood glucose levels drop at the start of exercise, these changes are small and short-lived and are corrected within 30 minutes of exercise. The benefits derived from carbohydrate consumption before an event are in fact greater than avoiding food prior to competition. However, individuals with pre-existing hypoglycaemia or diabetes mellitus should experiment, since they may benefit from trying out low GI foods, manipulating the time of the pre-event meal or using carbohydrates during the event.

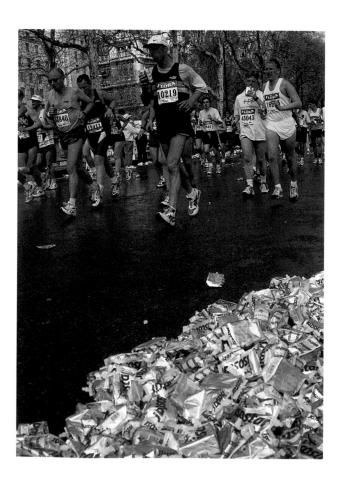

NUTRITION DURING COMPETITION OF MORE THAN 30 MINUTES' DURATION

PRINCIPLES

Carbohydrate (provided either by food and/or drink) and fluid need to be ingested during exercise, especially if the event is longer than 30 minutes. This is necessary to maintain blood glucose levels and ensure adequate hydration without causing any discomfort in the gut. About 30–60g carbohydrate per hour should be consumed. The maximum that the body is able to oxidize is 60g carbohydrate per hour. Medium to high glycaemic index (GI) carbohydrates are the best choices. Since the rules and conditions of certain sports may limit the opportunities to eat and drink, each athlete needs to look for the opportunities and establish a carbohydrate and fluid plan during exercise.

Tips

- Use carbohydrate-rich drinks and compact carbohydrate sources (bars, gels, sweets) together with sufficient fluid to meet your carbohydrate requirement of 1g per minute (60g per hour).
- In longer events or extreme activities such as ultra-endurance triathlons you might want to include solid food. Still focus on high-carbohydrate, low-fat options.
- During competition fluid intake is important to prevent dehydration. Use every opportunity to drink fluid such as injury time and half-time. Familiarize yourself with your own fluid requirements in different environmental conditions (*see Fluid, chapter 4*).
- Carbohydrate and fluid ingestion during shorter events or races is not practical nor is it necessarily a limiting factor. However, for athletes who participate in many events on the same day (for example, 100m sprint heats and finals) and for participants in multiday events, a recovery plan is critical.

RECOVERY
[POST-COMPETITION AND POST-TRAINING]

PRINCIPLES

Recovery nutrition should replenish liver and muscle glycogen stores, replace fluid and electrolytes lost in sweat, and regenerate and repair damaged tissue. There is a window period after exercise when the rate of glycogen synthesis is optimal. You should take 1–1.5g high GI carbohydrate per kilogram of body weight within 60 minutes after exercise and at frequent intervals until the next meal. Adding a small amount of protein will stimulate carbohydrate storage and result in faster repair and recovery of muscles. This is important if you lack appetite or have a short recovery period.

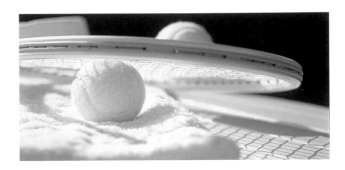

Opposite *Carbohydrate requirements can be met during exercise with sports drinks, bars and gels.* **Bottom** *Recovery snacks providing 50g carbohydrate and more than 10g protein.*

Tips

- Replace carbohydrate, fluid and electrolytes (sodium and potassium) within 30 minutes after exercise. A small amount of protein could be included.
- For every hour that you train, choose 1–2 of the recovery snacks, depending on your body mass. If you weigh more than 80kg (176 lb), opt for 2–3 recovery snacks. This can be a combination of fluid or solid foods, depending on your appetite and whether you are competing again in the next 1–2 hours.
- If there is more than 30 minutes between training and the next meal, take portable snacks to training.
- Drink to a plan.
- Post exercise rehydration goals should be to replace any remaining fluid losses that may not have been made up during exercise as well as the continued losses that occur in the recovery period.
- Avoid alcohol and caffeine in the post-recovery period.
- In team sports a coordinated recovery approach is often helpful where the team/management organizes suitable snacks and drinks.

Recovery snacks

500ml (1pt) sports-specific recovery formula

250–350ml (½pt) carbohydrate energy drink + 250ml (1 cup) liquid meal supplement

200–300ml (1 cup) fruit smoothie/milkshake

250ml (1 cup) low-fat fruit yoghurt or 350ml (1½ cups) drinking yoghurt

200ml (1 cup) drinking yoghurt + low-fat energy bar

Small handful of lean beef jerky + low-fat energy bar or dried fruit bar

2 sports bars providing a total of 50g carbohydrate and 10–20g protein

Sandwich with low-fat cheese/cottage cheese/lean cold meat/chicken + 1 fruit

Bowl of cereal with low-fat or fat-free milk

30g (1 oz) lean beef jerky + 500–750ml (1–1½pt) carbohydrate energy drink or colddrink or fruit juice

30g (1 oz) lean beef jerky + 10 jelly babies + water

2 small packets pretzels or 6 rice cakes + 30g (1 oz) lean beef jerky/low-fat cheese

500ml (2 cups) instant mashed potato prepared with low-fat or fat-free milk

410g (14 oz) tin low-fat rice pudding

TRAVEL

While travelling there are many situations that are likely to challenge your nutrition plan. These challenges can include:

- delays in transit
- long-distance travel and jet lag
- hotel food
- budget constraints and limited food availability
- official functions (cocktail parties)
- foreign menus with unusual food choices
- standards of food hygiene
- interference with usual routines
- menu fatigue and boredom
- holiday atmosphere

You may be able to manage some of these challenges, but consulting with a sports dietitian ahead of travelling can eliminate these stressors and will ensure optimal nutrition when it's needed most.

JET LAG

When one crosses multiple time zones a new set of times is imposed on the body, which may conflict with the built-in circadian rhythm, giving rise to jet lag. This will occur whether one travels from east to west or vice versa, but is more significant when travelling west to east, and seems to affect older persons more severely.

Jet lag symptoms are very different to the tiredness and general discomfort (travel fatigue) that one feels after a long journey. Both conditions occur simultaneously, but travel fatigue generally resolves within 24 to 48 hours, whereas recovery from jet lag can take a lot longer. For instance, when travelling eastward from South Africa to Australia, it can take up to 11 days to recover; whereas travelling westward from Australia to South Africa may take half the number of days to recover.

Typical symptoms of jet lag include fatigue during the new daytime; inability to sleep at night; difficulty concentrating on tasks; irritability; disorientation and mental confusion;

headaches; loss of vigour; a loss of appetite coupled with indigestion and even nausea; change in normal bowel activity – constipation is common. Clearly these will have a negative effect on performance.

Behavioural, drug and dietary strategies can be effective in reducing the symptoms of jet lag. Behavioural strategies will include adjusting sleep patterns, exposure to natural light, timing of exercise and meals, etc. The use of certain drugs (sleeping tablets and melatonin) may aid adjustment, but should be discussed with a sports physician, since they can also have detrimental side effects.

Certain dietary interventions and the use of specific foods also assists adjustment.

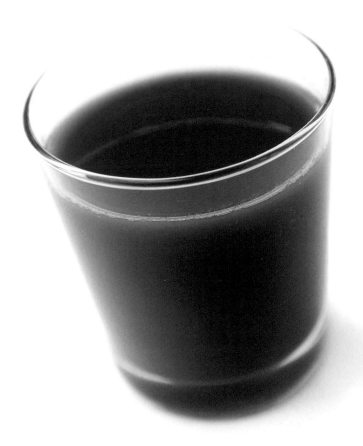

BEFORE THE FLIGHT

- In the week before departure, work toward adopting destination times for meals.
- Eat a high-protein breakfast with caffeinated beverages and then switch to caffeine-free, carbohydrate-rich foods/drinks (these have sedative properties) for the afternoon and evening meals and snacks.
- Pre-arrange all meals and snacks taken in transit.
- Pack into carry-on baggage some portable carbohydrate-rich snacks (higher-fibre options like breakfast and dried fruit bars, fresh and dried fruit, wholewheat crackers), sports bars, liquid meal/snack replacements, and sports drinks.

DURING THE FLIGHT

- Avoid alcohol, tea and coffee. Consume plenty of fruit juice, tomato juice, water, non-fizzy cordials and sports drinks instead.
- The last meal prior to the time allotted for sleep should be high in carbohydrate and low in protein. This will induce sleep.
- On waking, to help raise the level of arousal and prevent a relapse into sleep, a high-protein breakfast with coffee/tea can be consumed.

UPON ARRIVAL

- Increase total fluid intake and time the intake of caffeinated beverages (e.g. coffee/tea/colas) to coincide with periods of high arousal.
- Evening meals and snacks should be high in carbohydrate (pasta, potatoes, rice, breads, vegetables, fruit, low-fat dairy drinks/desserts).

Opposite *Fruit juices are not only hydrating, as opposed to dehydrating drinks like coffee or alcohol, but are also rich in antioxidants. Tomato juice contains the antioxidant lycopene.*

Travel tips

- You need to be clear about your nutritional goals to stay committed while travelling and avoid temptation to eat whatever comes your way.
- Investigate the food at the destination ahead of time.
- Find out about food hygiene and water safety in the countries you are to visit and avoid high-risk foods (the skin of unpeeled fruit and unbottled water).
- Take supplies with you if important foods are likely to be unavailable or expensive. Foods that are portable and low in perishability include: liquid meal formulae, carbohydrate powders, sports drinks, breakfast cereals and instant oats, dehydrated foods, skim milk powder, dried fruit and fruit sticks, pretzels, microwave popcorn, low-fat quick-cooking noodles, sports bars, crackers, plain biscuits, sweets, chocolate powder, yeast (vegetable) extract and beef jerky (if allowed to be brought into the country).
- Special meals and menus in restaurants, aeroplanes or hotels can often be organized in advance.

SUPPLEMENTS

Supplements should not be used to replace healthy eating habits, but there may be situations where supplements may make a practical difference to your diet or performance. Supplements should only serve to enhance an already optimum nutrition game plan. There are many considerations, which include cost, safety and efficacy, which are covered in chapter 7.

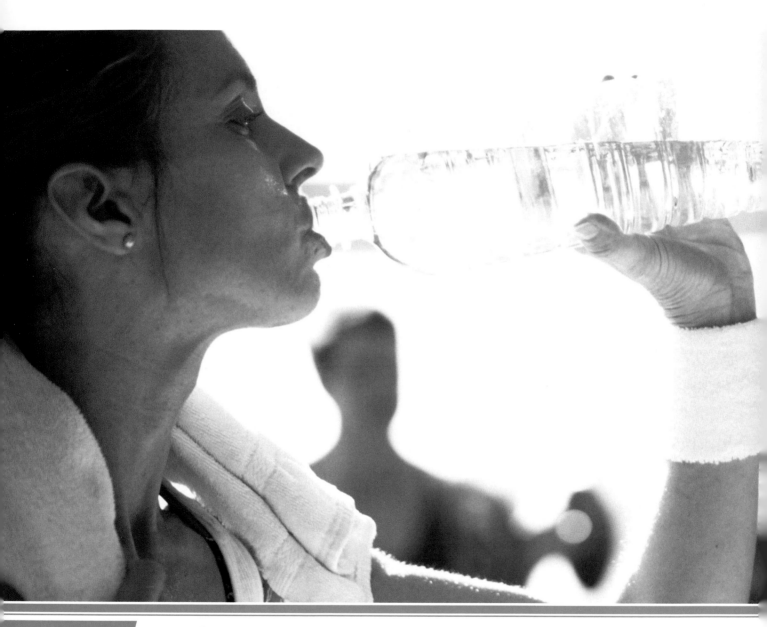

chapter 4

FLUID AND HYDRATION

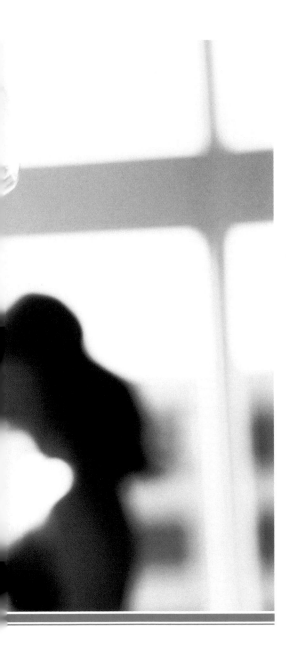

THE IMPORTANCE OF FLUID

Fluid plays a significant role in optimizing your sports performance, regardless of your type of sport. Research shows that athletes who do not drink anything during exercise will perform less well than they would if they drank *ad libitum* (according to thirst). This 'ad lib' recommendation must, however, not be interpreted as drinking as much as possible, since this has not been shown to improve performance and may even result in overhydration with serious consequences. The 'ad lib' approach, although not rigid and quantified, does still mean working to a plan and understanding the practical issues that may influence fluid accessibility in different sports.

The exact fluid requirement for different athletes is currently being debated. It is extremely difficult to measure the effects of fluid on sports performance, since there are so many different determinants; and studies up to now have not been consistent in the measurement of outcomes. Previous guidelines have not entirely been based on evidence and have incorrectly assumed that:

- ☒ all weight lost during exercise needs to be replaced
- ☒ thirst is not an accurate marker of fluid requirements
- ☒ fluid requirements are similar for all athletes, so a universal guideline is possible
- ☒ high rates of fluid intake can do no harm
- ☒ heat stroke is always a result of dehydration.

Furthermore, many studies have been done in controlled laboratory environments, whereas results may vary considerably on the field. Fluid requirements may also differ remarkably between athletes and between exercise situations. The type of sport, including duration and intensity as well as other factors such as sex, body size and composition, genetics and fitness, environmental conditions and clothing will all affect an individual's fluid requirements.

THE TYPE OF SPORT, INCLUDING DURATION AND INTENSITY

Duration and intensity of exercise will determine requirements. The same athlete may have different fluid requirements depending whether he or she is training or competing. Swimmers may train for 4–5 hours a day and incur great fluid losses, whereas in a 100m sprint event it is unlikely that dehydration will be a limiting factor.

Different individuals participating in the same race will have different requirements. According to the American College of Sports Medicine (ACSM) fluid guidelines of 1996, one should consume 150–300ml (0.3–0.6pt) every 15 minutes. However, these guidelines are currently being challenged because they do not consider the slower athlete participating in ultra-endurance events, who may be at risk of overconsumption of fluids.

Deliberate dehydration techniques to 'make weight' are commonly practised in weight-category sports. When giving guidelines to athletes participating in these types of sports, one has to take into consideration the conventional wisdom or lore of the sport, the rationale and the consequences of these practices. The use of saunas, sweat suits, vigorous exercise, and/or the use of diuretics (banned substances) are some of the strategies used in a desperate attempt to make weight. Even with these extreme practices, the effects of dehydration on strength in these types of sports are difficult to assess and may depend on the time and strategies used to rehydrate before competing.

HOW GENETICS AND FITNESS AFFECT FLUID REQUIREMENTS

Some athletes sweat more than others and fitter people start sweating earlier in exercise and in larger volumes. Trying to match these fluid losses with larger fluid intakes may not, however, translate into better performance as the winning athletes in prolonged events have been shown to be the most dehydrated!

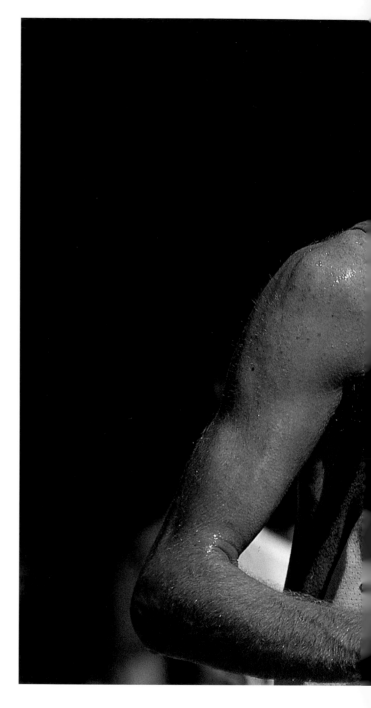

SEX, BODY SIZE AND COMPOSITION

In general, women lose less sweat than men performing the same workload. This is because of a lower average body weight and a greater percentage of body fat for the same weight as men. Adipose (fat) tissue is about 10% water,

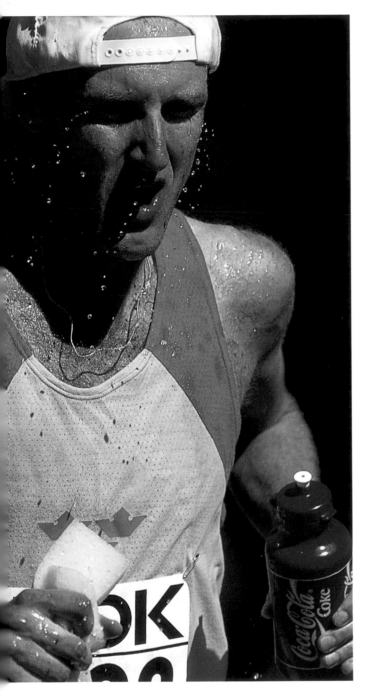

ENVIRONMENTAL CONDITIONS AND CLOTHING

In hot climates, the perception of effort is increased, and exercise capacity is reduced. The mechanisms responsible for the reduced exercise performance in the heat are not entirely clear, but it is proposed that a high core temperature is involved. This theory is based on the observation that a period of acclimatization is successful in delaying the point of fatigue, but this occurs at the same core temperature. The primary effect of acclimatization is to lower the resting core temperature. Altering body heat before exercise can alter exercise capacity. In other words, performance can be extended by prior immersion in cold water and reduced by prior immersion in hot water.

Uniforms, protective gear and strapping also have a profound effect on sweat loss. Persons wearing protective garments often have a sweat rate of 1–2 litres per hour (2–4pt/hr) during light-intensity exercise. For many team sports, with rules and uniforms more appropriate for cooler climates, it is important that players take cognizance of increased fluid requirements when playing or competing in hotter environments, and modify their clothing accordingly.

There are also certain practicalities and features unique to different sports that can affect fluid intake. Tailoring a fluid plan to suit your individual needs is discussed in the sports-specific chapters of part 2 (chapters 8 to13). This chapter provides general guidelines and practical strategies on fluid recommendations before, during and after exercise.

compared to muscle tissue's 75%. Therefore individuals with more muscle have a greater water reservoir and are less affected by dehydration. Body composition therefore determines an athlete's ability to overcome the detrimental effects of dehydration.

Left *The 'nothing new' rule: practise your fluid replacement strategies when training to determine your requirements under different conditions.*

THE ROLE OF FLUID
THE PHYSIOLOGY OF HYDRATION

The continual regulation of the volume and composition of body fluids is essential for optimal body functioning. This regulation involves the relationship between the external environment and the body, as well as the interchange taking place between the body's own cells, tissues and organs. Normal osmotic pressure, nerve function, muscle contraction, the movement of nutrients into cells and the removal of waste from cells is dependent on electrolytes and non-electrolytes held in solution. The regulation of electrolytes, in turn, is closely tied to that of water.

Water is the main solvent of the body. It provides the medium for biochemical reactions within cell tissues. It is essential for maintaining blood volume, acid-base balance, kidney and heart function as well as the regulation of body temperature.

When a person exercises, total body metabolism is typically increased to 5–15 times the resting rate. Approximately 70–90% of this energy is released as heat, which needs to be dissipated to achieve body heat balance. In hot climates a substantial volume of body water can be lost via sweating to enable evaporative cooling. Some electrolytes are also lost through sweat. By replacing both fluid and electrolyte losses you can avoid the effects of dehydration.

THE RISKS OF DEHYDRATION

- Increased core body temperature; the body begins to overheat.
- Strain on the heart as the heart rate increases for a given workload due to the increased viscosity of blood.
- Perceived effort is greatly increased and concentration, skills and mental functioning are diminished.
- Rehydration is much more difficult to achieve because of the subsequent gastrointestinal discomfort and upsets.

SIGNS

Early signs of dehydration are: headache, fatigue, loss of appetite, flushed skin, heat intolerance, light-headedness, dry mouth and eyes, urine is dark and has a strong odour.

Advanced signs of dehydration require urgent medical attention. These are: difficulty in swallowing, clumsiness, shrivelled skin, sunken eyes and dim vision, painful urination, numb skin, muscle spasms and delirium. Intravenous therapy may be required.

FLUID AS A SOURCE OF OTHER NUTRIENTS

Carbohydrate replacement and fluid replacement offer different advantages to sports performance. The combination of carbohydrate and fluid improves performance, meaning that these effects are both independent and additive. This makes a strong case for trying to meet both fluid and carbohydrate requirements during exercise, but these do not always follow the same formula.

In some sports events, the athlete has large sweat losses (fluid) with a smaller need to replace fuel (athlete who has dehydrated to make weight), whereas in other sports events, the athlete may deplete fuel stores without losing great amounts of sweat.

Sports drinks typically have a carbohydrate concentration of 7%, which provides 50g of carbohydrate when consumed at an hourly rate of 700ml (1½ pt) of fluid, which will meet the requirements of most athletes. Individuals may want to change the total volume (for instance, larger athletes in hotter environments may need to drink more) and the ratio to favour the balance that suits the specific needs of their event (*see The Ideal Drink pp65–67*).

Opposite *Examples of carbohydrate-rich drinks and their uses.*

IMMUNITY BENEFITS

Recent studies have shown that regular fluid consumption during exercise also has immunity benefits. Saliva contains several proteins with antimicrobial properties. These include IgA, lysozyme and alpha-amylase. Saliva secretion usually falls during exercise, but if fluid is consumed, saliva flow rate and the secretion of saliva IgA can be maintained. This may have particular significance for endurance athletes who may be more susceptible to upper respiratory tract infections after major events.

TYPE	VOLUME (ML) TO PROVIDE 50G CARBOHYDRATE	COMMENTS
Sports drinks (5–8% carbohydrate + electrolytes)	600–1000ml (1–2pt)	Designed for athletes to provide carbohydrate and fluid and small amounts of electrolytes
Concentrated sports drinks (>10% carbohydrate + electrolytes)	330–500ml (⅔–1pt)	Useful for carbo-loading and during some ultra-endurance events; but may provide insufficient fluid during an event and increase the risk of gastric discomfort
Soft drinks and cordials (10–11%; very low sodium)	500ml (1pt)	May be more slowly absorbed due to the higher carbohydrate content; useful for a taste change but then may need to be diluted; some contain caffeine
Designer energy drinks (11–12% carbohydrate + guarana, ginseng, taurine, caffeine)	450–500ml (≈ 1pt)	No electrolytes; herbal substances are not regulated; consider the risks and benefits of caffeine and guarana in sport
Fruit juices (8–13% carbohydrate; may have added vitamins and minerals; low sodium)	385–625ml (¾–1¼pt)	Negligible source of electrolytes; carbohydrate may be more slowly absorbed; risk of diarrhoea if juice is high in fructose
Flavoured sports drink powders and concentrates (contain carbohydrates and electrolytes)	Volume varies according to carbohydrate concentration	Useful as you are able to vary the concentration according to your individual fluid and carbohydrate requirements
Sports gels (60–70% carbohydrate + electrolytes and may contain vitamins and caffeine)	1½–2 sachets	Concentrated carbohydrate source but provides no fluid which still needs to be met (with water); experiment to determine tolerance as it can cause gastric discomfort

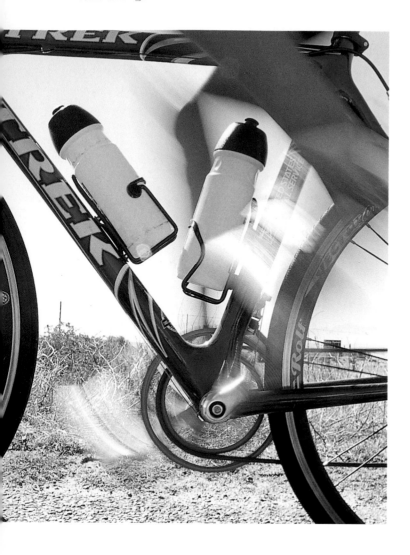

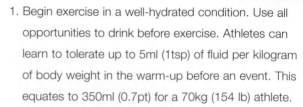

Tips

1. Begin exercise in a well-hydrated condition. Use all opportunities to drink before exercise. Athletes can learn to tolerate up to 5ml (1tsp) of fluid per kilogram of body weight in the warm-up before an event. This equates to 350ml (0.7pt) for a 70kg (154 lb) athlete.

2. Use a fluid replacement plan that has been practised in training. Drink as much as is practical and comfortable in attempting to match sweat losses. Note that even when exercising in water or in air-conditioned venues, sweat losses will be incurred. Start drinking early and top up frequently as this will maintain gastric volume and increase fluid absorption.

3. The drink must be cool (not cold), palatable and contain the optimal amount of carbohydrate for your event.

4. Make the most of opportunities to drink (stoppages, injury time in team sports).

5. Make sure that your drink is readily available, not in the change rooms. It should be in a container that allows easy drinking with minimal interruption of exercise.

6. Replace fluid losses as completely as possible between competition sessions. Note that after exercise you will continue to lose sweat for some time. Fluid replacement after exercise is assisted by the simultaneous replacement of electrolytes (sodium and potassium). *(See pp65–67.)* Make active cooling part of your recovery plan. Do not spend a long time in a hot tub or spa and, if you do, drink extra fluid.

7. When fluid deficits are greater than 1.5–2l (3–4pt) and the time for rehydration is short, rehydration solutions (used to treat diarrhoea) with a sodium content of 60–80mmol/ℓ *(see glossary)* can be used. Pretzels, soup or potatoes dipped in salt, taken with water, are also good sources of sodium.

8. Fluid intakes of children, the elderly, pregnant and lactating athletes are discussed in chapter 2.

GENERAL FLUID GUIDELINES AND TIPS

Dehydration during exercise is usually the result of a mismatch between thirst and fluid requirements. Athletes may also drink little to avoid weight gain or to avoid urinating during the event. Of course, the rules of the sport and stoppages as well as the availability of fluids during the event may also affect fluid practices. Here are some general tips that will encourage good fluid practices for all athletes.

Above *Ensure that your drink is readily available in training and competition.*

CAN YOU EVER DRINK TOO MUCH?

RISKS OF OVERHYDRATION

Hyponatraemia (low blood sodium levels) can occur in ultra-endurance events lasting longer than four hours as a result of the overconsumption of fluid diluting the body's sodium levels (less than 130mmol/ℓ). Slower athletes, overzealous with their fluid consumption, are especially at risk.

Avoid overhydration by:

- being sensitive to the onset of thirst as the signal to drink, rather than 'staying ahead of thirst'
- ensuring adequate salt intake in the fluids consumed
- having salty snacks before, during and after exercise
- monitoring weight – weighing more after training than before is a sign of developing water intoxication
- being aware that non-steroidal anti-inflammatory drugs and pain relievers can contribute to developing a water overload.

SIGNS OF OVERHYDRATION

Nausea, vomiting, extreme fatigue, respiratory distress, dizziness, confusion, disorientation, oedema (rings, watches and shoes may feel tight), coma, seizures and even death if left untreated.

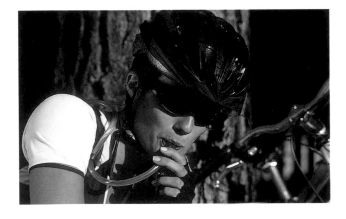

Above *'Camelbacks' make fluid easily accessible, but avoid overhydration by 'trying to stay ahead of thirst'.*

THE IDEAL DRINK

Sports drinks are specially formulated to meet the dual aims of carbohydrate and fluid delivery, with palatability being another important feature.

CARBOHYDRATE
TYPE AND AMOUNT [CONCENTRATION]

The amount of carbohydrate in the drink (concentration) can be varied according to individual needs and environmental and climatic conditions. When carbohydrate needs are more important, a higher carbohydrate concentration not exceeding 10% or 60g carbohydrate per hour will be of benefit. Greater concentrations delay gastric emptying and may cause diarrhoea and stomach cramps and may even increase the risk of dehydration. In events lasting longer than 30 minutes, carbohydrate-containing drinks have been shown to enhance performance more than plain water. However, in extremely hot conditions, when fluid needs take priority, a more dilute solution of 4% carbohydrate (containing sodium) can be used.

Preference should always be given to drinks containing glucose or glucose polymers. Glucose polymers (called glucose syrups and maltodextrins) are obtained from the partial digestion of cornstarch and can provide as much as 10 times the energy of the simple sugars for the same osmolality (*see p66*) without slowing the rate of gastric emptying. Glucose polymers consist of a number of glucose molecules, which are joined together, resulting in a lower osmolality than if the same solution consisted of unlinked glucose molecules. Unflavoured glucose polymers have no taste and are therefore useful in situations where extra carbohydrate is required without added sweetness.

Fruit juice during exercise is not recommended as fructose delays gastric emptying and so decreases the rate of fluid absorption. Furthermore, excessive fructose may increase the risk of diarrhoea and gastric upset.

What about Osmolality?

Sports drinks are often marketed on the basis of their osmolality, although it should not be your only consideration (the amount of carbohydrate is probably more important). Osmolality is a measure of the number of particles in a solution (concentration). In a drink these particles will be carbohydrate, electrolytes, sweeteners and preservatives. In blood plasma the particles will be sodium, proteins and glucose. Blood has an osmolality of 280–330mOsm/kg (*see glossary*).

Drinks with an osmolality of 270–330mOsm/kg are in balance with the body's fluid and are called isotonic. Hypotonic fluids have fewer particles than blood and hypertonic fluids have more.

The osmolality of a drink determines which way the fluid will move across a membrane (the gut wall). If a drink with a high osmolality is consumed, then water moves from the bloodstream and gut cells into the gut, resulting in net secretion (temporary dehydration). If a drink with a low osmolality is consumed, then water is absorbed from the gut (the drink) into the gut cells and bloodstream, resulting in net water absorption.

Hypertonic solutions are absorbed at a slower rate than hypotonic or isotonic solutions, thus delaying the desired hydration and energy benefits. During training or competition, hypertonic solutions can also have a dehydrating effect as your body draws on its available fluids to dilute the solution down to an isotonic level. Hypotonic solutions are therefore more effective when rapid rehydration is desired and is suitable for athletes such as golfers who need fluid without the boost of carbohydrate. Isotonic or hypertonic drinks are more beneficial in events where energy demands are high, such as ultra-distance events.

A drink with a 10% glucose solution will have a higher osmolality than a drink with the same carbohydrate concentration, but made up of glucose polymers (which will not affect the sweetness).

ELECTROLYTE COMPOSITION AND CONCENTRATION

Sodium and potassium, the main electrolytes lost through sweat, are found in limited amounts in most commercial sports drinks. A carbohydrate-containing sports drink containing 52mmol/ℓ sodium and 25mmol/ℓ potassium would be ideal, but too much sodium affects the taste of the drink and so the amount of sodium in drinks (10–30mmol/ℓ) only partially replaces the sodium lost in sweat (ranging from 10 to 90mmol/ℓ).

Electrolyte replacement during ultra-endurance events is even more important and the use of salt pills may be of benefit, especially on a hot day. Foods and snacks with a high salt content can also help make up these losses.

The sodium concentration in sweat averages 35mmol/ℓ (the range is 10–70mmol/ℓ) and varies according to diet, sweat rate, hydration and degree of acclimatization (acclimated persons have up to 50% lower sodium sweat concentrations for any specific sweat rate).

There is a low risk of running into deficiencies of potassium, magnesium or calcium during exercise. Potassium may need to be replaced after exercise.

OTHER ACTIVE INGREDIENTS

Always check the labels of drinks for any other substances, some of which may be counterproductive or even banned.

VITAMINS AND MINERALS

Sports drinks generally need not contain vitamins, since losses via sweat are low. Optimal intakes of vitamins and minerals should still be met in the diet.

CAFFEINE

Caffeine and caffeine-like substances may be present in some drinks. Caffeine has a diuretic effect and should be avoided in the post-exercise recovery period. However, during exercise it does not increase urine production. As of 2004, caffeine is no longer considered a banned substance. Previously, a urinary caffeine concentration above 12µg/ml was considered as doping. This concentration could be achieved by consuming 500mg of caffeine in a short period (although this would have varied between individuals). Sources of caffeine include coffee, tea, some sports bars and gels, and chocolate bars (see p156).

GLYCEROL

There has been some interest in adding glycerol to hydration beverages in order to enhance fluid retention and maintain a relative hyper-hydration prior to and during exercise. Glycerol can be taken orally in the form of commercially available glycerine solutions. Special hyper-hydration supplements are now being marketed to athletes. Glycerol is a 3-carbon molecule similar to alcohol. It occurs naturally in the body as a component of stored fat and a small amount is present in body fluids as free glycerol. While some studies have observed enhanced exercise performance with glycerol ingestion, others have not. The mechanisms are unclear, with potential negative consequences such as weight gain, headaches, gastrointestinal distress, nausea and blurred vision. It is therefore premature to recommend glycerol hyper-hydration.

SPORTS WATER – JUST ANOTHER GIMMICK?

Sports waters are uncoloured, lightly flavoured drinks that contain electrolytes and are quickly gaining popularity. Sports water has fewer calories than sports drinks, and has more nutrients than water. Since sports waters are lightly flavoured, many athletes prefer the taste compared to that of the more strongly flavoured sports drinks. Flavour preference changes when the body is working hard and it is important to ensure that whatever fluid you choose is palatable during exercise. If the flavouring in sports water appeals to you during exercise and encourages you to drink more, this is a positive feature. Sports water is useful if your exercise session is less intense (not limited by carbohydrate) or if you are cutting back on your energy intake.

Practical tips

1. Allow for adequate recovery and rest after training.
2. Keep hydrated during exercise – but don't overdo it.
3. Sports drinks (5–7% concentrations) are a good option since they empty from the stomach more quickly than soft drinks (generally 10% concentration), while also helping to replace sodium losses. Drinks greater than 10% may promote gastric cramps.
4. Adopt a pattern of drinking small amounts of fluid at regular intervals during exercise rather than trying to drink large volumes all at once.
5. Eat salty foods – sandwiches with yeast (vegetable) extract, pretzels, beef jerky and salty crackers.
6. Follow the pre-match eating guidelines (see p53).
7. Breathe with the diaphragm, strengthen the abdominals, and stretch progressively. Increasing the intensity and duration of your training gradually will also help prevent stitches and cramps.
8. You can ease a stitch by slowing down or reducing your intensity. Bend forward while pushing on the affected area and breathing deeply. Lie down while elevating your hips.

PALATABILITY

This includes flavour, taste, mouth-feel and temperature and may have a large impact on voluntary fluid intake. Drinks should be cool and palatable for the individual. Note that taste does change during exercise and if a drink is unacceptably sweet during or after exercise, experiment with other drinks or reduce the concentration and add unflavoured glucose polymer powders.

CAN WARM DRINKS BE CONSUMED WHEN EXERCISING IN THE COLD?

Yes, as long as the drink is at a temperature that can be consumed. Warm drinks do not delay gastric emptying and do not have a negative effect on thermoregulation. They may also give a psychological boost to athletes undertaking events in cold climates.

CRAMPS AND STITCHES

Scientists are still trying to find out the exact cause of these two conditions and how to avoid them.

A cramp is a sudden, tight, intense pain that most commonly occurs in the leg muscles and is caused when the muscle contracts and does not relax. Cramps are a temporary event and usually do not lead to serious problems. Should they be severe or occur regularly or fail to improve with simple treatment, you need to see a doctor.

Factors that contribute to cramping may include poor fitness (tired muscles), exercising at high workloads, too little stretching, dehydration, especially when sodium losses are high, and creatine use (as reported by athletes who use it). Potassium, magnesium or calcium deficiency as a cause of cramps does not have much scientific support.

A stitch is a localized pain usually felt on the side just below the ribs and usually eases a few minutes after stopping exercise. As with cramps, the exact cause is unknown. During exercise it is possible that a full stomach contributes to a stitch. Eating and drinking inappropriately may also

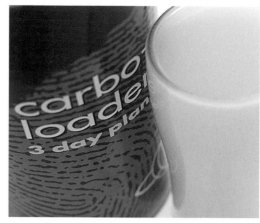
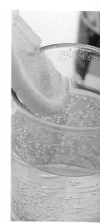

aggravate a stitch. Drinking or eating too closely to exercise, eating fatty foods, drinking fluids with too high a sugar concentration (because they empty slowly from the stomach), and dehydration may all be contributing factors.

ALCOHOL

Alcohol reduces reaction time and impairs balance, accuracy, hand-eye coordination, strength, power, endurance and body temperature regulation. After exercise alcohol interferes with the recovery of carbohydrate stores and acts as a diuretic, thereby aggravating dehydration. Alcohol also has a vasodilatory effect, which can increase bleeding and swelling, thus delaying recovery and healing. Specific sporting codes prohibit the use of alcohol in competition.

Opposite *Energy and alcohol content of various drinks (340ml = 1 can; 25ml = 1 tot; 120ml = 1 wine glass).*
Above from left *Sports drinks add carbohydrate and electrolytes; avoid alcohol 24 hours before an event; low fat milk is a valuable source of protein, carbohydrate and calcium.*

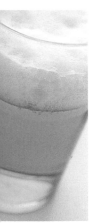
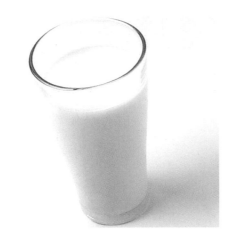

BEVERAGE	VOLUME	ENERGY	ALCOHOL (G)
BEER			
Alcohol free	340ml (11 fl oz)	234kJ (55kcal)	–
Average	340ml (11 fl oz)	584kJ (140kcal)	10
Lager	340ml (11 fl oz)	575kJ (137kcal)	10
Pilsner	340ml (11 fl oz)	483kJ (115kcal)	10
Cider	340ml (11 fl oz)	598kJ (143kcal)	10
SPIRITS			
Brandy, Cane, Gin, Vodka, Whisky	25ml (≈1 fl oz)	261kJ (62kcal)	10
Liqueurs	25ml (≈1 fl oz)	352kJ (84kcal)	10
Cream liqueurs	25ml (≈1 fl oz)	341kJ (81kcal)	10
Muscatel, Port	50ml (≈2 fl oz)	286kJ (68kcal)	10
Sherry (dry & medium), Vermouth	50ml (≈2 fl oz)	223kJ (53kcal)	10
WINE			
Red, Rosé, White, Semi-sweet	120ml (≈4 fl oz)	357kJ (85kcal)	10

Tippling tips

1. Stick to the 24-hour rule – avoid alcohol in the 24 hours before a competition and during multiday matches (some teams ban alcohol consumption).

2. After training or competition, you should first rehydrate and refuel with carbohydrates – ensure that plenty of nonalcoholic drinks are available.

3. Alcohol should be avoided if you have any soft tissue injuries or bruising.

4. Note that although some alcoholic beverages do contain carbohydrate (beer, for instance) the alcohol content of the drink affects performance, so you should rather resort to other, more appropriate, sources of carbohydrate.

5. Alcohol intake can be reduced by:
   - plenty of ice in spirit drinks – this dilutes the alcohol while increasing the volume, so you drink less
   - quenching your thirst with nonalcoholic beverages first (mineral water, fruit juice or a colddrink), so that the alcoholic drink is not used as a thirst quencher
   - ordering mineral or soda water with the alcohol
   - choosing low alcohol wines or beer.

6. Remember that soft drinks, fruit juices and mixers increase the energy content of alcohol. While drinking alcohol you also tend to eat more.

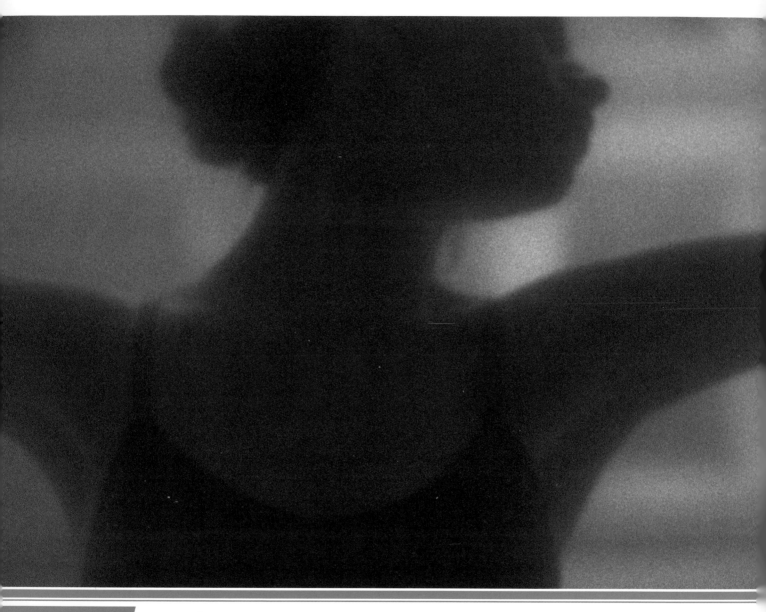

chapter 5

DISORDERED EATING IN SPORT

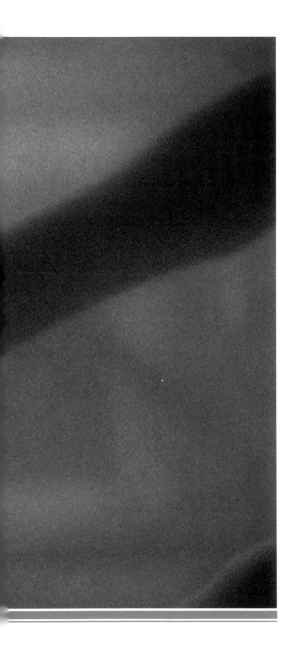

HARMFUL EATING BEHAVIOURS

Eating disorders (ED) are more prevalent among athletes than non-athletes and the incidence of ED and weight manipulation in athletes is probably higher than currently believed. In case studies done in the 1980s, anecdotal reports and press accounts mainly focused on females participating in aesthetic sports like gymnastics and ballet. Recent research has confirmed a high prevalence in elite athletes (including males), particularly in sports in which leanness or a specific weight are considered to be important.

Athletes who are at moderate risk of developing harmful eating habits may not necessarily show the symptoms of a full-blown ED, but even mildly harmful eating patterns can lead to health problems.

Disordered eating often involves a combination of harmful eating behaviours such as restricting food intake, the use of diuretics, laxatives and diet pills, self-induced vomiting and fasting. This may be associated with a strong preoccupation with food, compulsive exercise, distorted body image or a fear of weight gain. Although disordered eating in athletes may not be a clinical eating disorder – by not meeting the Diagnostic and Statistical Manual of Mental Disorders, Fourth Edition (DSM IV) criteria for anorexia or bulimia – it nevertheless includes some of the major symptoms of these diseases.

This chapter includes a list of causes and trigger factors, warning signs and extracts from the two best-known screening tools developed specifically to help in the diagnosis of eating disorders in athletes.

CAUSES AND TRIGGER FACTORS

[NOT IN ORDER OF IMPORTANCE]

1. Pressure to optimize performance and win at all costs. There are parents who 'surrender their children to sport'.

2. Meeting weight goals, through either prolonged periods of dieting or weight cycling, when competing in an inappropriate weight category, for instance.

3. Psychological factors and personality traits (poor coping skills, unhealthy family dynamics, low self-esteem, competitiveness, perfectionism, compulsiveness, high achievement expectations).

4. Large increase in training volume and significant weight loss associated with this. This could be the result of an early start to sport-specific training.

5. Injury and overtraining, causing changes in body weight.

6. Recommendation to lose weight without balancing this with guidance and support.

7. Comments and remarks made by coaches or staff, including public weighing.

8. Traumatic events including illness or injury to self or family member, new coach, leaving home, etc.

SCREENING TOOLS

The DSM IV may be used by clinicians together with other diagnostic criteria and measurements to confirm the diagnosis of an eating disorder. The warning signs tabulated here can be used to alert you that you may be at risk.

Two of the screening tools that have been developed for athletes are the FAST (Female Athlete Screening Tool) by McNulty *et al* and the SEDA (Survey of Eating Disorders among Athletes) by Guthrie *et al*.

The questions on the following pages are extracts from questionnaires devised by researchers to identify athletes at risk of developing eating disorders. They are given here only as a complement to the warning signs given below. They are not self-scoring tests, but are administered by qualified health professionals.

WARNING SIGNS OF ANOREXIA NERVOSA

- Dramatic weight loss
- A preoccupation with food, calories and body mass
- Wearing baggy or layered clothing
- Relentless, excessive exercise
- Mood swings
- Avoiding food-related social activities (refusing to eat with teammates)

WARNING SIGNS OF BULIMIA NERVOSA

- A noticeable body mass loss or gain
- Excessive concern about body mass
- Bathroom visits after meals
- Depressive moods
- Strict dieting followed by eating binges
- Increased criticism of one's body

ADDITIONAL WARNING SIGNS

- Amenorrhoea
- Stress fractures
- Hypoglycaemic symptoms during exercise
- Unexplained decrease in exercise performance
- Compulsive exercise
- Disturbed sleeping patterns
- Periodic bloating (due to refeeding or rehydration)
- Tooth decay, carotenaemia (yellow skin), lanugo (fine hair) on face and body, bloodshot eyes

Right *Warning signs of eating disorders.*

Opposite *Questions selected from the FAST screening tool.*

FAST (FEMALE ATHLETE SCREENING TOOL)

If I cannot exercise, I find myself worrying that I will gain weight.

① frequently   ② sometimes   ③ rarely   ④ never

I weigh myself

① daily   ② twice or more often per week

③ weekly   ④ monthly or less often

If I were injured, I would still exercise even if I were instructed not to do so by my athletic trainer or physician.

① strongly agree   ② agree

③ disagree   ④ strongly disagree

During season, I choose to exercise on my one day off from practice or competition.

① frequently   ② sometimes   ③ rarely   ④ never

My friends tell me I am thin, but I feel fat.

① frequently   ② sometimes   ③ rarely   ④ never

In the past two years I have been unable to compete due to an injury.

① seven or more times   ② four to six times

③ one to three times   ④ no significant injuries

I strive for perfection in all aspects of my life.

① strongly agree   ② agree

③ disagree   ④ strongly disagree

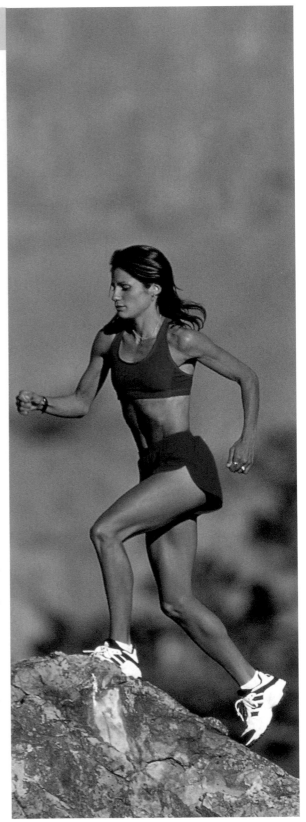

DIETARY SURVEY COMBINING QUESTIONS FROM TWO SCREENING TOOLS, AS USED BY DE PALMA et al

1) What is your current weight?

_____

2) Please circle on the scale below how much your eating behaviours interfere with the following:

Work	① Never	② Rarely	③ Sometimes	④ Often	⑤ Always
Daily Activities	① Never	② Rarely	③ Sometimes	④ Often	⑤ Always
Thoughts	① Never	② Rarely	③ Sometimes	④ Often	⑤ Always
Feelings about myself	① Never	② Rarely	③ Sometimes	④ Often	⑤ Always
Personal relationships	① Never	② Rarely	③ Sometimes	④ Often	⑤ Always
Extra curricular activities (sports, etc.)	① Never	② Rarely	③ Sometimes	④ Often	⑤ Always

3) How often do you weigh or measure your body size?

Ⓐ More than 3 times daily   Ⓔ More than weekly

Ⓑ 1–3 times daily   Ⓕ Weekly

Ⓒ More than daily   Ⓖ Monthly

Ⓓ Daily   Ⓗ Less than monthly

4) Certain factors within the athletic environment may contribute to the onset or development of eating patterns. Please indicate to what extent the following factors have contributed to your eating patterns on a scale from 0 (no contribution) to 4 (moderate contribution) to 10 (strong contribution).

_____ Ⓐ Weight loss was required for performance excellence

_____ Ⓑ Weight loss was required to meet a lower weight category

_____ Ⓒ Weight loss was required to meet aesthetic ideals

_____ Ⓓ A member of the athletic personnel (e.g. coach, trainer, sports psychologist) made a remark concerning my need to weigh less

_____ Ⓔ I had to be weighed in front of an audience (e.g. other team members)

_____ Ⓖ Each team member's weight was made public knowledge

_____ Ⓖ I was required to reduce my level of body fat in accordance with the coach's (or that of another member of the athletic personnel) desired ideal

_____ Ⓗ I was fearful of losing a position on the team or of being kicked off the team if I did not control or lose weight

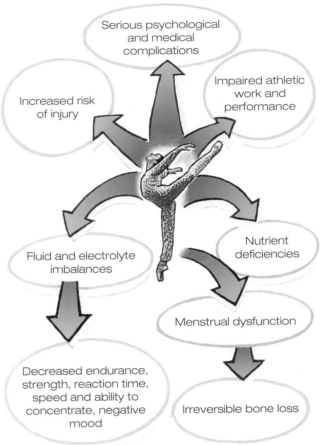

Serious psychological
and medical
complications

Increased risk
of injury

Impaired athletic
work and
performance

Fluid and electrolyte
imbalances

Nutrient
deficiencies

Menstrual dysfunction

Decreased endurance,
strength, reaction time,
speed and ability to
concentrate, negative
mood

Irreversible bone loss

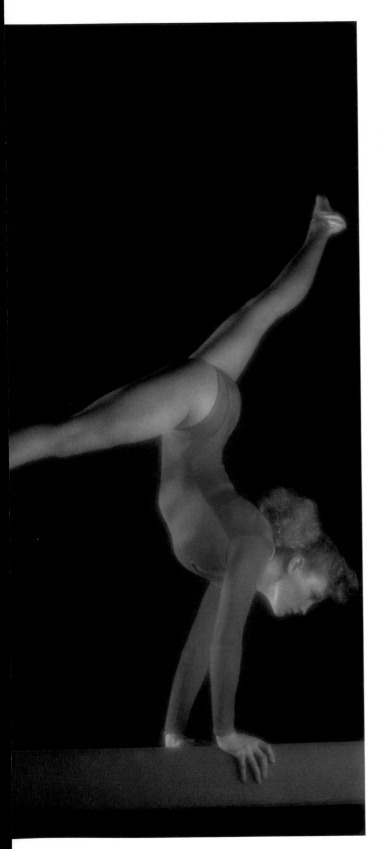

GET THIN AND WIN?

Much of the weight loss is due to loss of muscle tissue and this can affect training, which cannot be sustained with low levels of lean body tissue. Inadequate intakes of energy and nutrients will also limit the effectiveness of training. Dehydration from laxative use, diuretics and fluid restriction will significantly impair performance.

The restricted intake of a variety of foods may lead to medical complications which can be fatal, such as cardiac failure. Eating disorders may precipitate amenorrhoea and increase the risk of bone mass loss and stress fractures.

Above *Risks associated with eating disorders.*

THE FEMALE ATHLETE TRIAD

Female athletes can develop abnormal eating patterns (disordered eating), which can be associated with menstrual dysfunction (amenorrhoea or oligomenorrhoea) and subsequent decreased bone mineral density (BMD), or osteoporosis. These three conditions – disordered eating, amenorrhoea, and osteoporosis – often occur together in female athletes and have been termed the female athlete triad. Osteopenia is an early stage of osteoporosis.

Each of these disorders is of medical concern by itself, but when all three components are present, there is the potential for more serious effects on health, and also the risk of injury and death. The athlete, parents and coach should be made aware of the dangers associated with any of these conditions.

MENSTRUAL DYSFUNCTION

In the athlete, menstrual dysfunction is at least two to three times more common than in the non-athlete and is related to many factors, including a history of weight fluctuations, rigorous training schedules, an inadequate energy intake causing an energy drain, social pressures associated with competition and nutrient deficiencies.

Primary amenorrhoea is defined as the absence of menses by the age of 16. If menses have not occurred within four and a half years after the onset of breast development, clinical evaluation should be considered. Secondary amenorrhoea is typically defined as the absence of at least three to six consecutive menstrual cycles in a female who has begun menstruating.

It is incorrect to assume that amenorrhoea is a benign consequence of strenuous exercise. The altered hormone environment is a risk factor for the development of impaired bone health and osteoporosis.

Osteoporosis in the young female athlete refers to inadequate bone formation and also bone loss. This results in low bone mineral density and increased risk of bone fracture. Even if corrected with oestrogen replacement and calcium supplementation, the impact on bone health may be partially irreversible. Osteopenia is not as extreme as osteoporosis, but the risk of developing osteoporosis is determined by the peak bone mass achieved in adolescence and early adulthood.

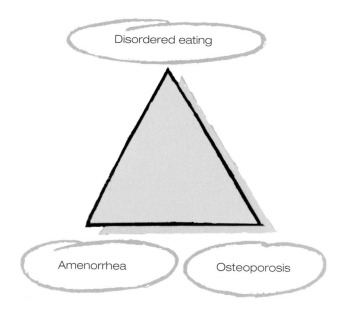

Above *A graphic depiction of the three cornerstones of the Female Athlete Triad.*

Right *The combination of low body weight, low body fat, poor nutrition and excessive training can lead to menstrual disturbances.*

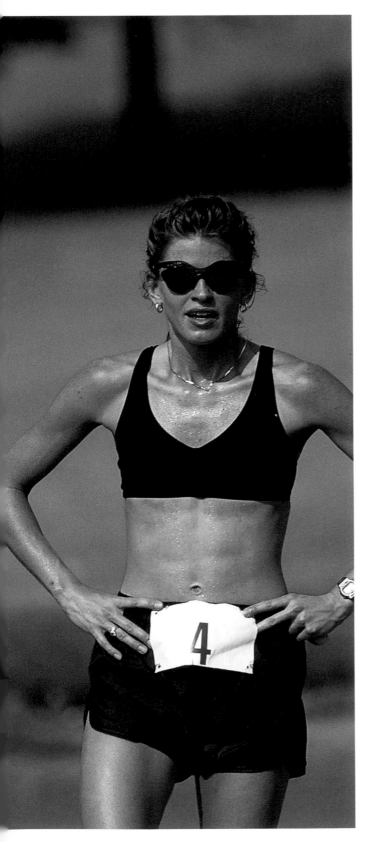

MANAGEMENT

- Treatment requires a multidisciplinary approach and even specialist treatment (gynaecologist, dietitian, psychologist). Regular medical assessment (blood tests, blood pressure, heart rate and body temperature) and monitoring of menstrual cycles is advised.

- Body composition rather than body mass should be monitored. It is difficult and potentially dangerous to define an ideal weight and/or percentage body fat for each sport or participant (*see p126*). Weight is not an accurate estimate of body composition, and when weight is lost, muscle and fat are lost. Weight gain should not be the focus of treatment unless the client is medically compromised.

- There must be consensus, rapport and trust between athlete, coach, selectors and parents. Neither punitive measures nor excessive praise should be part of the process. A process of negotiation is important.

- Interventions should be specific to the sport and the individual. It may not be necessary to stop exercise altogether, but the type and amount of exercise may need to be adjusted (for instance, by introducing one rest day a week and more weight training). However, an adolescent athlete with menstrual dysfunction may be required to gain weight before resuming athletic activity. More importantly, energy intake must be increased. However, this should be done gradually (taking into account the current energy intake and patterns of the athlete) so as to reduce the feeling of fullness that often increases the urge to exercise or purge. Start with 'safe' foods and progress to foods and eating situations that create less anxiety for the athlete. Nutrition education (for example, on the use and abuse of diet pills) may be needed.

- Supplementation with calcium (up to 1500mg/day) may be required, but this will only be effective if oestrogen levels are sufficient. In some cases low-dose oral contraceptives may be prescribed by a medical practitioner.

SPORTS ANAEMIA

Sports anaemia should not be confused with true iron deficiency. Sports anaemia is more common among female exercisers and is characterized by apparently reduced haemoglobin levels, but unlike true iron deficiency anaemia, performance remains unaffected. Although sports anaemia has a similar profile of iron status measures compared to iron deficiency anaemia, the red blood cells are normal in colour and size. A low iron status measure in athletes is thus not necessarily a true iron deficiency and can be a dilutional effect caused by the expanded plasma volume.

Sports anaemia (pseudoanaemia) occurs in athletes early in the training programme, especially after a rest period or injury or after an endurance phase of training. It is usually transitory and is sometimes treated unnecessarily with supplementation. Since it is difficult to differentiate between sports anaemia and true iron depletion, it is necessary to track and monitor iron status over a period of time.

True iron deficiency anaemia is found in athletes and untrained individuals alike, but more common in females. This condition reduces exercise capacity and negatively affects performance. Iron supplementation has side effects and should only be prescribed if an athlete is truly anaemic.

BIGOREXIA
BIGGER AND BETTER?

Bigorexia Nervosa, also known as muscle dysmorphia or the Adonis Complex, is characterized by the belief that the body is not lean or muscular enough, despite comments by others to the contrary (distorted body image). It is not an eating disorder, but an obsessive-compulsive disorder. *Rexia* means appetite, so both bigorexia (big appetite) and anorexia (no appetite) are misnomers. In the case of bigorexia it is a preoccupation with muscle size.

Sufferers may give up social, occupational and recreational activities to spend more time working out, often through illness and injury. They wear layers of clothing, avoid exposing their bodies and use substances such as steroids, food supplements and fat burners, even when they know the risks (*see p100*). Lowered libido (a side effect of steroid use) is exacerbated by physical exhaustion or self-consciousness to the point that they can no longer relax and enjoy sex. Depression may also be a feature of the condition.

Below *A graphic depiction of sports anaemia.*
Opposite *A high-energy diet with training is required to 'bulk up'.*

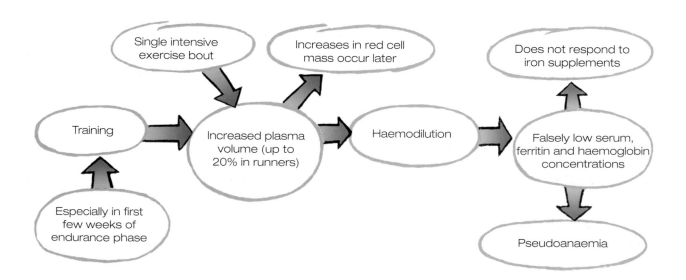

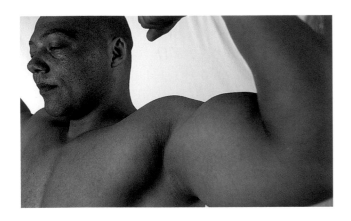

WHO IS AT RISK?

Specific screening tools have been developed, but it is still an under-researched area.

It is estimated that in America about 10% of all hard-core gym people have some degree of bigorexia. A study found that almost 54% of those interviewed at an amateur weight-lifting competition met the criteria for bigorexia. Body builders, wrestlers, gym trainers and TV stars (like those on *Gladiators*) would also be susceptible.

Men are more at risk than women. The media convey the idea that a six-pack (abdominal muscles), impressive pecs (pectoral muscles) and large lats (lateral back muscles) will improve their confidence, sex life and their sense of being in control.

Gyms are increasingly targeting women, for whom it used to be good enough just to be thin. In women, amenorrhoea and low levels of zinc and iron are additional concerns.

WHAT ARE THE EATING HABITS OF A BIGOREXIC?

The diet is usually very rigid, repetitive and monotonous with close monitoring of protein, carbohydrate and fat. Protein intake may be as high as 40% of total energy intake with plenty of egg whites, lots of chicken breasts, tuna (in brine), steak, and skim milk powder being consumed, sometimes with carbohydrate (rice cakes, rice or pasta). Specific combinations of foods are eaten together or only 'natural' foods.

Meals are also eaten frequently – every three hours and sometimes throughout the night, using an alarm clock.

Competitive body builders with bigorexia may alter their diet and cycle supplement intake depending on the phase of training or competition. In the muscle-bulking phase, this could mean a high-energy, high-protein diet (which may include protein supplements) with moderate carbohydrate, and then switching to a very low-energy, fat-cutting diet (that may include fat-cutters) in the few days before a competition. This is then followed with a high-carbohydrate, low-fluid (some even use diuretics), low-sodium diet to get 'ripped'. The whole sequence may then be followed by post-competition bingeing.

SHOULD ONE BE EATING HIGH PROTEIN, NO CARBOHYDRATES AND LOW FAT?

One should never exclude a particular food group, since this will always cause nutrient imbalances.

It is a myth that you need plenty of dietary protein to build muscle. Your muscles are only able to use a limited amount of protein for growth, provided there is enough carbohydrate to fuel the strength training required for your muscles to grow. Any excess protein (amino acids) will be broken down and either stored as fat or later used as a source of energy.

The process of breaking down amino acids also necessitates the excretion of water and thus excessive intakes of protein may compromise fluid balance. A consistently high protein intake may also contribute to kidney disease and gout and may accelerate calcium losses.

Even after training, when you need the extra protein to derive the anabolic and recovery benefits, this must be consumed with carbohydrate.

Current accepted recommendations on protein requirements for athletes fall within the range of 1–2.2g/kg body weight or as a percentage of total energy intake (15–25%). Fat requirements for athletes may be as low as 20% of total intake, with carbohydrate making up the balance.

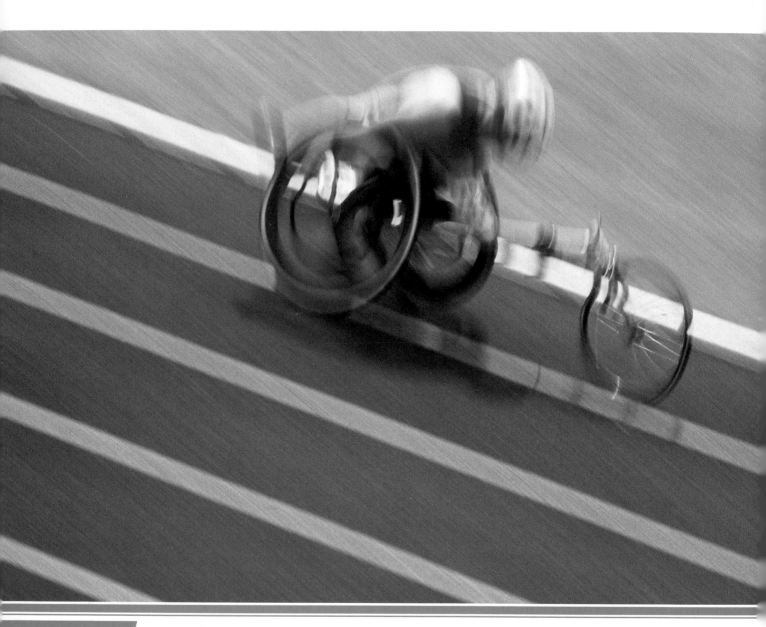

chapter 6

SPECIAL NEEDS AND MEDICAL CONSIDERATIONS

VEGETARIAN ATHLETES

Vegetarians may be classified according to the animal foods that they exclude. Lacto-ovo vegetarians exclude all animal foods except milk products and eggs. Lacto-vegetarians exclude all animal foods and eggs and vegans exclude all animal foods, dairy and eggs. A fruitarian diet is the most restrictive form of a vegetarian diet in that only raw fruits, nuts and seeds are eaten. The more restrictive the diet, the more difficult it is to achieve a balanced diet.

ENERGY

It may be challenging for vegetarian athletes to meet their energy requirements as the diet is usually high in fibre (bulky), making it difficult to consume large quantities of food. This is of special concern in children who need energy for growth and development. To maintain a high energy intake, spread food over six or seven meals throughout the day, include high-energy drinks such as fruit smoothies or liquid meal replacements and some less bulky carbohydrates like white bread and pastas.

PROTEIN

Protein requirements are more easily achieved when consuming animal foods. For instance, 90g (3 oz) chicken breast supplies the same amount of protein as 375ml (1½ cups) of cooked legumes. Moreover, protein from plant foods, with the exception of soya and tofu (soya bean curd), are incomplete because they lack some essential amino acids. The quality of the protein can be improved by combining vegetable proteins that complement each other. A vegetable protein food that contains a good supply of some essential amino acids, while lacking in one or two others, should be combined with a vegetable which provide the missing essential amino acids.

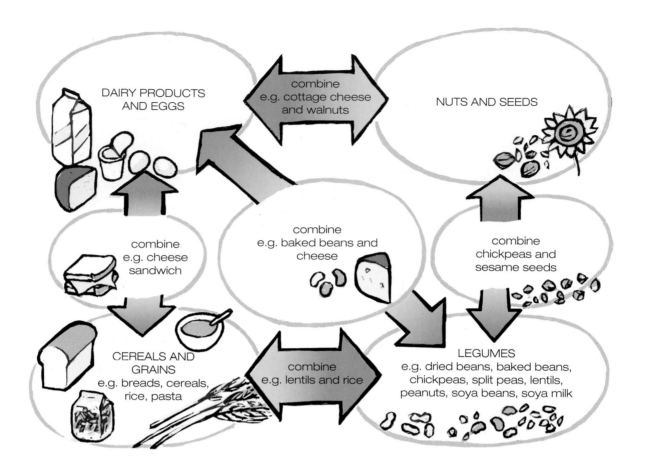

FAT

Not all vegetarian foods are low in fat. Nuts, seeds, cheese and certain processed soya products may contain a significant amount of hidden fats. However, the type of fat in these foods (except for the dairy foods) is generally poly- and monounsaturated and are better alternatives to the saturated animal fats.

CALCIUM, VITAMIN D AND B_{12}

When dairy products are avoided in the diet, it is more challenging to achieve adequate intakes of calcium, vitamin D and B_{12}. Fortified foods such as soya milk and breakfast cereals may provide these nutrients. However, vegans and older vegetarians who have less efficient B_{12} absorption may require vitamin B_{12} supplementation.

IRON

Iron from meat products is far more easily absorbed than the iron from plant foods. Including vitamin C (citrus fruits and drinks) with each meal will increase the absorption of iron from plant foods. Tannin (in tea), caffeine, and too much fibre will inhibit iron absorption.

Above *Protein from most plant foods lacks some essential amino acids; these foods need to be combined with others that supply the missing amino acids.*

CLASSIFICATION OF GIT SYMPTOMS IN ATHLETES	NUTRITION SOLUTIONS	RISK SPORTS INCLUDE
UPPER GIT		
■ Nausea and vomiting	Before exercise eat low-fat, low-fibre, easily digestible meals and snacks that empty from the stomach quickly	LOW RISK: swimming, cycling, running, triathlon MEDIUM RISK: aerobics, canoeing
■ Heartburn	Avoid highly concentrated carbohydrate beverages. Sip small volumes of drinks frequently. Avoid foods known to irritate (caffeine and fatty foods, chocolate and peppermint)	
LOWER GIT		
■ Abdominal cramp and urge to defecate	Consume a low-fibre and low-residue diet before exercise and avoid lactose-containing foods and drinks before exercise. Establish a routine of emptying the bowel before exercise	LOW RISK: cycling, swimming MEDIUM RISK: aerobics HIGH RISK: canoeing, running, triathlon
■ Diarrhoea	Eat a low-fibre, low-residue diet; or a diet high in soluble fibre (e.g. oats and oat bran; apple) consider anti-diarrhoeal drug therapy	

GUT PROBLEMS

There are several factors that contribute to gut problems during exercise. These can be as a result of physical trauma, dehydration, and changes in stress hormones, which decrease blood flow, disturb motility (movement of the bowel, or peristalsis), and alter the movement and absorption of food in the gut. A thorough diagnostic approach is necessary to exclude any pre-existing bowel diseases (such as Crohn's or coeliac disease) or other secondary causes such as drug use (anti-inflammatories, for instance). When travelling athletes need to practise safe eating and drinking habits (see pp56–57).

Above *Dietary solutions can help avoid gastrointestinal tract (GIT) symptoms during exercise.*

DIABETES MELLITUS

I am diabetic. Is it safe for me to exercise?

Exercise is beneficial for persons with Type I and Type II diabetes provided blood glucose levels are controlled. Exercise should be combined with diet and insulin or drug treatment. Diabetes is a condition in which there is a shortage of the hormone, insulin. It is produced by the pancreas and is responsible for the transport and uptake of glucose by the cells of the body. Exercise increases glucose uptake by the muscles, thereby helping to lower blood glucose levels. Exercise will also improve the sensitivity of the body to insulin. It helps to reduce body fat and reduces the risk of diabetic complications. Exercise is not recommended if your blood glucose levels are not controlled, in which case it may aggravate symptoms.

Do I need to adjust my diet when I exercise?

The recommended goals and guidelines are no different to those for athletes without diabetes. Your training diet should include carbohydrate-rich foods with a low glycaemic index (GI) (see opposite) and low-fat foods, which are compatible with diabetes management and athletic performance. Rather than change your eating to suit your drug or insulin dosages, make adjustments according to your training regime. Consistent training and eating routines promote good diabetes management, so it is best to exercise at the same time each day in order to fine-tune your regime.

You will also need to consider the timing of meals and snacks as well as the insulin dose and its predicted peak period of activity in relation to the exercise routine. It is critical that you monitor your blood glucose levels regularly to assist in the adjustment of food and insulin to prevent and manage hyper- and hypoglycaemia.

In general, the recommended carbohydrate intake before, during and after exercise is no different to that for the athlete without diabetes, assuming good metabolic control and that blood glucose levels are between 4 and 8mmol/ℓ (80–160mg/dl). Blood glucose levels on either side of this

range may require adjustments to food intake. If blood glucose levels are too low, additional carbohydrate is required. If blood glucose levels are higher than 14mmol/ℓ (280mg/dl), ketones need to be checked and exercise may need to be postponed until your blood glucose is within recommended ranges. You will have to monitor your blood glucose frequently and adapt these carbohydrate recommendations on the basis of your own response to exercise depending on the intensity, duration and type of exercise, which is often a process of trial and error.

How do I prevent hypoglycaemia (low blood glucose levels)?

Avoid exercising during periods of peak insulin activity. If using short-acting insulin, inject in the abdomen rather than the exercising limb and reduce the dose if necessary. Follow the dietary recommendations outlined above and always ensure that you train with a partner who is familiar with the symptoms of hypoglycaemia. Have a quickly absorbed carbohydrate (high GI) available. To prevent late hypoglycaemia after exercise, you may need to reduce the next insulin dose. A further risk associated with hypoglycaemia is impaired temperature regulation, so adequate hydration is essential for optimum performance.

Note that alcohol is also a factor for late hypoglycaemia as it blocks gluconeogenesis (the biosynthesis of glucose from non-carbohydrate precursors in the liver) and it can mask the symptoms of hypoglycaemia.

What causes hyperglycaemia (high blood sugar levels) during exercise?

Infection, the overconsumption of food or highly concentrated sports drinks (usually for fear of the onset of hypoglycaemia), inadequate insulin and, in some cases, alcohol consumption.

Should I carbo-load before an endurance event?

Use this strategy with caution. This regime is dependent on the availability of insulin to store muscle glycogen. You may also need to adjust your insulin dose to match the changes in your diet, as well as the tapering effects of exercise before a competition.

Note: it is advisable for athletes with diabetes to work in close consultation with a sports physician and dietitian, especially when newly diagnosed.

Below *Glycaemic index is a ranking of the effect on blood glucose of eating a single food relative to a reference carbohydrate (glucose, in this table). If the GI of baked potatoes is 85, that means it produces a rise in blood sugar 85% as great as when eating an equivalent amount of glucose.*

GLYCAEMIC INDEX (GI OF SELECTED CARBOHYDRATE FOODS
GI VALUE (GLUCOSE = 100)

HIGH GI (70 AND ABOVE)	INTERMEDIATE GI (55–69)	LOW GI (BELOW 55)
Glucose	Grapenuts	High-fibre breakfast cereal
Most sports drinks	One-minute oats	Muesli, toasted
Corn-based breakfast cereal	Oat porridge	Special K
Cocopops	Oat bran (raw)	Wheat (whole kernel)
Crisped rice cereal	Muesli (not toasted)	Barley
Shredded wheat	Rye bread	Bulgur
Instant mashed potato	Pita bread	Fructose
Baked potato	Taco shells	Banana (under-ripe)
French fries	Muffins	Cherries
Maize meal porridge	Crumpets, pancakes	Grapefruit
Rice cakes	Soft drinks and cordials	Grapes
Melba toast	Orange juice	Orange
White bread	Sucrose (sugar)	Peach (fresh)
Wholewheat bread	Popcorn	Pear
Breakfast wheat biscuits	Ice cream	Baked beans
Rice noodles	Banana (over-ripe)	Butter beans
Watermelon	Mango	Chickpeas
Honey	Raisins	Kidney beans
Rice (low amylose)	Baby new potatoes	Lentils
Pumpkin	Beetroot	Soya beans
Pretzels	Brown rice	Spaghetti
Jelly beans	Basmati rice	Macaroni
	Couscous	Instant noodles
		Green peas
		Sweet potato
		Seed loaf
		Low-fat plain yoghurt and sugar-free yoghurt

Note: *The GIs of porridge and cereals differ from country to country.*

DISABILITIES
ENERGY REQUIREMENTS AND WEIGHT GAIN

The daily energy expenditure of athletes with disabilities can be as much as 30% lower when confined to a wheelchair. Energy intake will need to be adjusted accordingly and the focus should be on nutrient-dense foods low in fat and sugar.

FLUID REQUIREMENTS

The practical consequences of consuming adequate fluid require more attention in athletes with disabilities. The recommended volume, frequency and type of fluid remain the same, provided the gut function is unaffected. Other practical factors that need to be considered when planning a fluid regime include proximity to toilet and water facilities.

When exercising in the heat, active cooling (in shade), spraying with water and applying cooling devices may be needed. In cold environments, active heating and heat-loss prevention may be required.

FIBRE

Constipation is very common, especially if mobility is limited or gastrointestinal damage has occurred. Dietary fibre intake together with adequate fluid and frequent meals are important to help regulate bowel movements.

MEDICATIONS

It is important to be familiar with the potential side effects of medications that are frequently used as they may affect dietary recommendations.

Opposite top *Infection risk is reduced at low to moderate exercise workloads but increases at higher workloads (from Nieman et al. 1990).*
Opposite bottom *An athlete with burn out suffers fatigue inappropriate to the workload.*
Below *Careful planning is needed to ensure that disabled athletes have easy access to food and fluid at training and competition venues.*

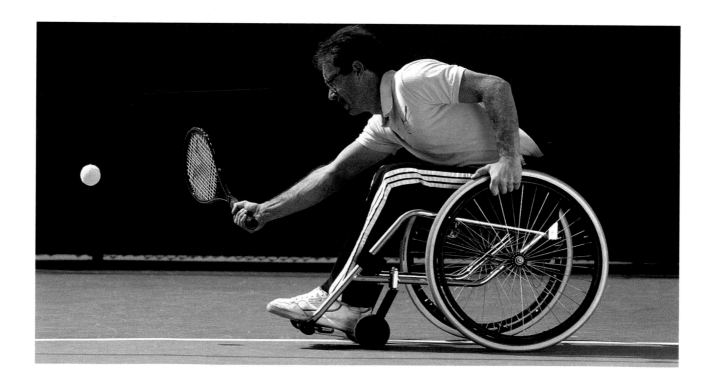

CHRONIC FATIGUE
UNEXPLAINED UNDERPERFORMANCE SYNDROME

There is a reason why the Arabs have 23 words for desert, the Inuit have 23 words for snow and exercise scientists have 23 words for overtraining.

'*The roots of overtraining seem as diverse and dim as the definitions, and the consequences range from muscles to motivation.*' – R Eichner, 1995

When the fatigue experienced is inappropriate for the amount and intensity of training, and performance deteriorates, the athlete may be suffering from chronic fatigue. It may be caused by overtraining, viral illness, upper-respiratory tract infection, decreased immunity, inadequate nutrition, eating disorders, insufficient sleep, psychological stress, anxiety or depression. There are of course many other medical causes of chronic fatigue, including metabolic disorders, cardiac problems, allergic disorders, infections, malignancies and anaemia.

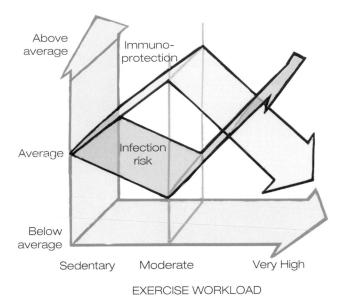

SIGNS AND SYMPTOMS OF CHRONIC FATIGUE:

■ fatigue and unexpected sense of effort during training

■ frequent minor infections

■ unexplained or unusually stiff and/or sore muscles

■ mood disturbances

■ changes in expected sleep quality and patterns

■ loss of energy

■ loss of competitive drive

■ loss of libido

■ loss of appetite

■ excessive sweating.

To diagnose chronic fatigue in athletes, other medical conditions need to be excluded. A sports physician, psychologist or dietitian can use questionnaires to help identify any overt nutritional and lifestyle factors. One of these is called HEADS (Home, Education, Activities, Drugs & Depression, Sex and Sport), and the other, POMS (Performance of Mood States).

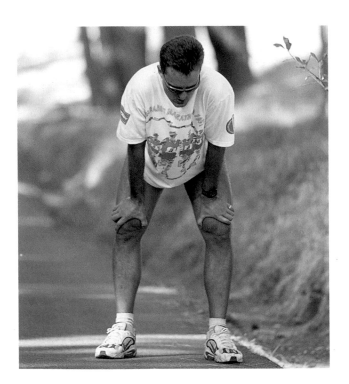

CHRONIC FATIGUE

Nutrition has great potential in the prevention and treatment of chronic fatigue. It is unlikely that a single nutritional factor is responsible for chronic fatigue, and more than one contributing factor needs to be addressed.

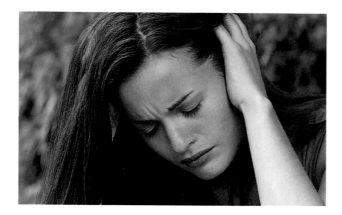

LOW ENERGY INTAKES

Energy needs of athletes range from 8360 to 25,080kJ/day (2000 to 6000 kcal/day) and sometimes even more. Meeting these higher energy intakes is often a challenge, considering the combined constraints of training, sleep, work and other commitments. If the diet is chronically very low in fat and high in carbohydrate, the task is even more daunting.

Under-eating and a low body mass is commonly seen in athletes with chronic fatigue. In female athletes, energy intakes of 5225 to 8987kJ/day (1250 to 2150kcal/day) have been associated with amenorrhea, frequent injuries, irritability, inability to concentrate, depression and poor athletic performance (*See p76*). If you do not eat enough you will not be getting all the macro- and micronutrients you need. Athletes with poor energy intakes frequently have poor vitamin and mineral intakes. Furthermore, chronic low energy intakes alter hormones such as leptin (a protein hormone with important effects in regulating body weight, metabolism and reproductive function) and thyroid hormones (which affect development, growth and metabolism), and these diminished levels may directly suppress immunity.

CARBOHYDRATE

If inadequate carbohydrate is consumed, repeated days of training lead to depletion of the muscle glycogen stores and fatigue. Carbohydrate has also been shown to have several immune-protective benefits, and may also counter glutamine depletion (*see section on glutamine below*).

Carbohydrate consumption during exercise has been found to reduce central fatigue by affecting the free tryptophan to BCAA ratio (*see Branched Chain Amino Acids p99*).

PROTEIN

Consistently inadequate protein intakes will not only affect muscle regeneration after exercise, and muscle growth, but will also lead to micronutrient deficiencies (iron and zinc) which, over time, will suppress immune function and increase the susceptibility to opportunistic infections.

As discussed in chapter 3 (Recovery), combining some protein with carbohydrate in the post-exercise period helps to build muscle and hastens recovery.

GLUTAMINE

Glutamine is a non-essential amino acid, because it can be synthesized by various tissues such as the skeletal muscles, liver, and adipose tissue. During exercise or at other times of metabolic stress (fasting, severe injury, illness), the demand for plasma glutamine increases. Various cells of the immune system, such as the lymphocytes and macrophages, depend on glutamine as a primary fuel source. However, studies of the effect of glutamine supplementation on performance and immune status showed conflicting results. More conclusive data is needed on the use of nutrition strategies (such as carbohydrate supplementation) that may counter glutamine depletion.

Above left *There are many nutritional factors that contribute to chronic fatigue.*

Oxidative stress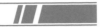

Free radicals are molecules that are created by your body through normal activities including digestion and respiration. Due to their chemical structure (a free radical lacks an electron), they are very unstable. So they seek out other molecules to steal electrons from them, which starts a chain reaction of molecular damage. This process is known as oxidative stress. If you have an elevated level of free radicals and not enough antioxidants to balance them, cellular damage results.

BRANCHED CHAIN AMINO ACIDS (BCAA)

High serotonin levels suppress appetite and cause sleepiness. High-volume training may result in chronic elevations of serotonin levels, which can explain some of the signs and symptoms of chronic fatigue. Studies in which the diet was supplemented with carbohydrate and/or BCAAs showed that serotonin levels can be altered. However, the effects on performance are unclear, possibly because the studies could not show small changes. Also, the increased production of ammonia associated with BCAA supplementation can have detrimental effects (*see p99*).

FAT

The type (the ratio of the essential fatty acids, omega 3 to omega 6) and total amount of fat in the diet may affect immune function. High- and low-fat diets alike have been associated with decreased immune function.

MICRONUTRIENTS

Micronutrients play an important role in energy production, haemoglobin (iron) synthesis, maintenance of bone health (calcium), and adequate immune function (zinc).

ANTIOXIDANTS

Strenuous physical exercise induces oxidative stress, which may overwhelm the body's antioxidant defence system. These defences include the antioxidant vitamins C and E and thiol antioxidants. Although some studies have shown that trained athletes may have increased antioxidant enzymes in muscle tissue, there is also evidence that antioxidant supplementation can help. The use of mega-doses of antioxidants can, however, be counterproductive and cause other health complications.

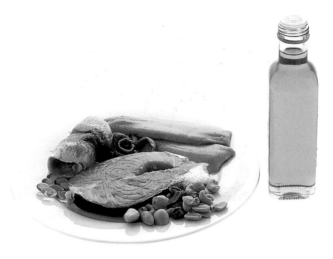

IRON, ZINC, SELENIUM

Deficiencies in zinc, iron and selenium may diminish the body's antioxidant defence system. Athletes who eat high-carbohydrate and high-fibre diets, or diets with little haeme iron (found in meat, fish and poultry), may have a poor intake of these minerals, especially in a bio-available form. However, excessive intakes of iron and zinc should be avoided as they have been shown to impair immune function.

Above *The quality and quantity of fat may affect immune function.*

OTHER, INCLUDING HERBAL PRODUCTS AND NUTRACEUTICALS

There are a number of nutraceuticals such as proanthro-cyanidins, plant sterols and sterolins which support the immune system. Also called phytochemicals or functional foods, they are natural, bioactive chemical compounds.

Examples are garlic, astragalus, ginseng, black seed (black cumin or Kalangee) and echinacea. The echinacea species (*Echinacea augustifolia* and *purpurea*) or Purple Coneflower has been shown to benefit athletes in at least one published study. Ginseng has been classified as a harmonizing agent, or adaptogen, often used by athletes to increase stamina and performance and to relieve stress. However, there are no published studies with conclusive evidence for its immune benefits (*see chapter 7*).

GUIDELINES IN THE USE OF THESE PRODUCTS

- It is best not to use these products continually for more than two or three months. The theoretical concern is that in certain conditions, prolonged enhancement of immune function may have an adverse effect, especially with regard to autoimmune illnesses like rheumatoid arthritis, multiple sclerosis, tuberculosis and HIV/AIDS.

- Topical preparations of echinacea should not be used by persons allergic to the daisy family of plants.

- Not much is known about the bioavailability of these products in supplement form, so the focus should be on dietary sources.

- Products containing herbs and adaptogens or nutraceuticals may contain ephedrine or other banned substances. Athletes have tested positive for ephedrine when taking a ginseng preparation.

- These products are not well controlled and manufacturing standards may vary (*see p94*).

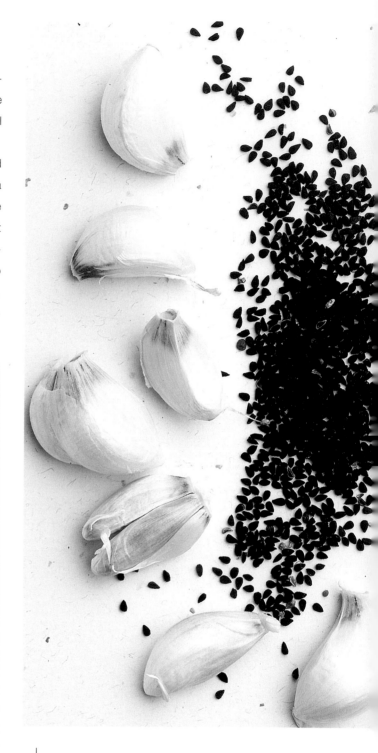

Above *Many natural, bioactive chemical compounds found in plants may be useful to the immune system.*

MANAGEMENT OF CHRONIC FATIGUE

GENERAL TIPS

- Avoid prolonged training sessions. Long-duration exercise sessions can be split into two shorter bouts, which may reduce the risk of immuno-suppression experienced following a single bout of prolonged exercise.
- Do not train with a fever.
- Include recovery days in your weekly training programme.
- Vary training to avoid monotony.
- Get adequate sleep.
- Monitor mood, fatigue and muscle soreness.
- Avoid sick people.
- Practise good personal hygiene.
- Avoid getting a dry mouth and don't share drinks bottles.
- Be aware of vulnerability/susceptibility after training or competition.

Below *Nutritional management of chronic fatigue.*

NUTRITIONAL PROBLEM	SOLUTION
Low energy intakes	- Weight should be appropriate to support training - Smaller, frequent meals and snacks that complement training schedules - All foods should be nutrient-dense - Supplement (over and above the diet) with a meal-replacement formula
Low carbohydrate intakes	- Match your carbohydrate intake to your training needs (*see chapter 1*) - During training include 30–60g carbohydrate/hour - Consume carbohydrate drinks during and after prolonged exercise - Use compact, low-fibre carbohydrate if appetite is lacking – e.g. fruit yoghurt, fruit juice, jam, honey, glucose polymer powders or gels, and low-fat sports bars
Low protein intakes	- Larger portions of lean protein at meals and snacks (e.g. beef jerky, tuna, chicken, low-fat cheese, eggs, hummus, tofu, quorn, beans and lentils) - Enrich milk-based foods and drinks with skim milk powder (add this to porridge, soup, mashed potatoes, smoothies) - See that your recovery snack also includes protein (*see p55*) - Use higher protein shakes to supplement the diet, but exercise caution with some sports brands (*see p98*)
Low fat intakes	- Include 20–30% fat in your training diet, limiting saturated fat to < 10% - Regularly consume foods rich in omega 3 fatty acids (mackerel, herring, halibut, salmon, green leafy vegetables, legumes)
Poor micronutrient intakes (vitamins and minerals)	- Avoid the indiscriminate use of these supplements - If dietary intakes are poor, correct the diet and use a multivitamin and mineral supplement if necessary - Supplement individual vitamins and minerals only on the advice of a sports dietitian or physician
Other (herbs, sterols, etc.)	- First optimize the diet before taking any of these supplements, taking the safety and efficacy of these products into consideration

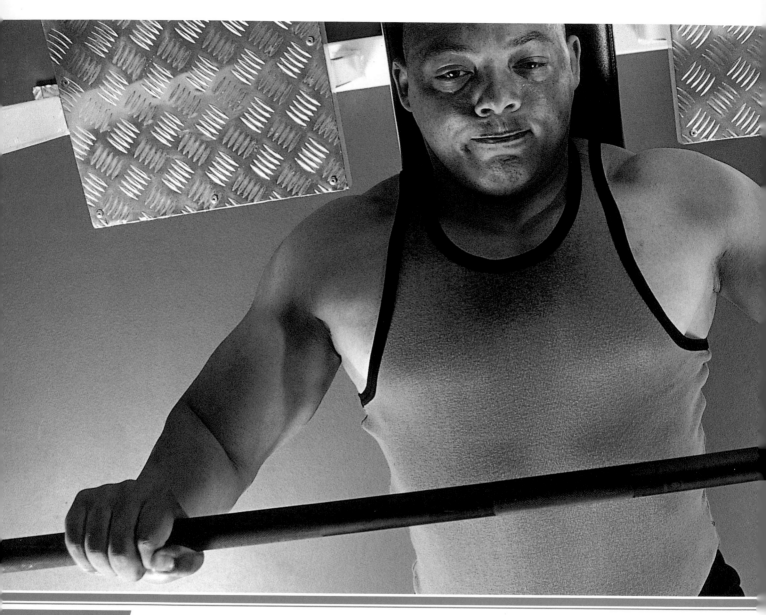

chapter 7

DIETARY SUPPLEMENTS

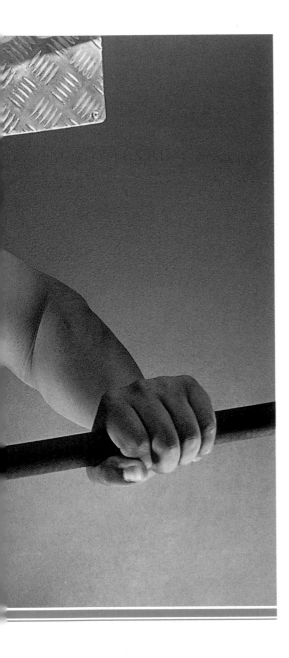

PERFORMANCE-ENHANCING, OR ERGOGENIC, AIDS

The desire to win by going faster, higher, stronger (the Olympic motto is *Citius, Altius, Fortius*) motivates athletes to look for anything to improve performance. In the case of nutrition, ergogenic aids refer to supplements that contain nutrients or food chemicals in amounts greater than would be found in dietary sources and are purported to have a direct supra-physiologic or drug-like effect on performance. This raises many questions.

The first question is an ethical one. The World Anti-Doping Agency (WADA) deems a substance or method to be on the List of Prohibited Substances and Methods if it meets any two of the following criteria:

- medical or other scientific evidence that the substance or method has the potential to enhance sports performance
- represents an actual or potential health risk to the athlete
- use of the substance or method violates the spirit of sport as described in the WADA code.

Substances or methods are also included if WADA determines there is medical or other scientific evidence that it has the potential to mask the use of other prohibited substances and methods.

You should also consider the health implications. Many supplements are sold on the premise of being powerfully beneficial, but also harmless. Surely, if a substance has such powerful effects then it should be regarded as a drug! However, since the adoption of the 1994 Dietary Supplement Health and Education Act by the US Congress, supplements have been specifically exempted from evaluation for safety and efficacy by the US Food and Drug Administration (FDA). Although there are some guidelines to the type of claim that can be made, the claims do not require FDA approval. According to this act, supplements are defined as any product (other than tobacco) intended to supplement the diet and contains one or more of the following ingredients: a vitamin, mineral, amino acid or metabolite; a herb or other botanical constituent; a concentrate, extract or combination of any of these ingredients, that cannot be represented as a conventional food. So, unlike registered drugs, which are tightly regulated, there is currently no proper control on the production, importation, distribution and marketing of supplements. There is no control on the exact composition of these products and there is no system to ensure that the products are safe and effective.

There is increasing evidence that some products may not contain the amount and proportions of the ingredients listed on the label, may not contain the ingredient at all and may even contain substances (toxins, contaminants or Schedule 4 and 5 substances) that can lead to significant health problems and, in the case of an athlete, a positive doping test (*see p96*). It is extremely difficult for athletes to separate false claims from facts.

The worldwide use of nutritional supplements by all athletes, including the elite, appears to be increasing and the survey done on Olympic athletes at Sydney shows astonishing results (*see above, right*). The aggressive marketing of sports supplements not only targets the elite athlete, but also often

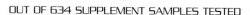

OUT OF 634 SUPPLEMENT SAMPLES TESTED

94 (14.8%) contained substances not labelled that would result in a positive doping test. Of these 94 samples, 23 contained banned pro-hormones (building blocks), which metabolize to both nandrolone and testosterone in the body. In addition to these 94 samples, 66 others (10.4%) returned borderline results for various unlabelled substances.

2758 OF THE 10,300 ATHLETES TESTED FOR DOPING WERE QUESTIONED ON THEIR USE OF SUPPLEMENTS

- 569 reported nil use in 3 days before being tested
- Vitamins were used 1996 times:

    880 times as individual vitamins; 73 times by injection

    1116 times as multivitamins (+ extra supplements); 17 times as injections

- Minerals were used 499 times (253 times as multiminerals)
- Proteins were used 18 times

    Amino acids were used 396 times (50 times as injections)

    Creatine was used 316 times (11 times by injection)

    HMB (beta-hydroxy beta-methylbutyrate) was used 24 times

- Herbal extracts were used 345 times (95 times as ginseng)
- 1 athlete took 25 separate items on one day

uses sporting celebrities to promote the use of these products to the general fitness enthusiast and young aspiring athlete. The demand for and supply of supplements is on the increase. As consumers become more concerned about their health, physical appearance as well as preventing and treating certain diseases, supplement companies are providing more and more product options (combinations of vitamins, minerals and herbs) that are heavily marketed and promoted, but not always supported by scientific research.

Above *Findings on the use of supplements by athletes at the Sydney Olympics, 2000 (B Corrigan, R Kazlauskas).*

Left *Findings of a 2001 International Olympic Committee study on supplements used by athletes.*

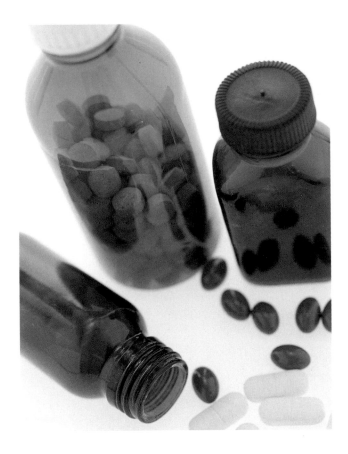

SUPPLEMENT RISKS VERSUS BENEFITS

It is unlikely that supplements will ever be able to replace the value of a well-planned sports-specific diet. An appropriate eating regime remains the foundation of a nutrition game plan, together with other factors vital for peak performance discussed in chapter 1. Supplements can be used in certain situations to fine-tune or top-up an already optimal diet (hence the word 'supplement' not 'substitute'). Specific supplements, if used correctly in certain situations, can play a small but useful role in performance and could be the difference between winning and losing.

WHY FOOD FIRST?

- Many foods and fortified foods can be used as supplements without all the risks and expense associated with supplements. For example, skim milk powder is a good, economical source of protein, carbohydrate and calcium, and can be added to enrich or fortify different foods. Breakfast bars are another example of a real food that is practical, portable and a good source of nutrients.
- Foods contain thousands of compounds that may be biologically active, including hundreds of natural antioxidants, carotenoids, and flavonoids.
- There are nutrient-nutrient interactions within the matrix of food, which may affect health.
- The bioavailability (absorption and metabolism) of nutrients is generally greater in food than in supplements.
- Compared to supplements or drugs, there is no risk of toxicity or of exceeding the Upper Limits (ULs).
- Supplements are often expensive.

Already in 1998 it was estimated that the annual sales of dietary supplements in the USA totalled $13.9 billion with 29,000 available products.

Supplements are easily available in health shops, gyms, pharmacies, via the Internet, as well as from health professionals who are targeted by companies and offered incentives to promote or sell their products.

We have used the most recent scientific evidence to evaluate the potential benefits versus the risks.

Above *Supplements should only be taken when there is evidence that the diet cannot provide the quantities of the nutrient needed.*

WHO SHOULD TAKE SUPPLEMENTS?

A thorough assessment of your current diet is needed to establish any nutrient deficiencies. This should also take into account body composition goals, dietary and medical history, gastrointestinal condition, eating patterns and food preferences, training and competition nutrition requirements, budget constraints, medications and stress.

Certain biochemical markers may be used to confirm findings from the dietary assessment, but they have limitations. The loss of nutrients during exercise is generally transient and physically active persons adapt to the effects of training in many ways: for example, increased plasma volumes may affect iron levels (causing pseudoanaemia). The value of some popular methods (such as analyzing hair samples) may not reflect current status (affected by shampoos and swimming pool chemicals, for instance).

If your diet is adequate, supplementation is unlikely to improve performance. Athletes whose diets are deficient in certain nutrients, vegetarians, athletes participating in aesthetic sports and following restrictive diets, athletes eating chronic high-carbohydrate diets, ageing athletes, athletes with medical problems and athletes exercising in extreme environments will require supplementation. However, a general multivitamin and mineral supplement, providing not more than 100–150% of the Recommended Dietary Allowance (RDA), would benefit most sportspersons and there may be certain situations (travel or injury, for instance) when it is practical to use a short-term supplement. Supplements that will make a practical difference to the diet include meal replacement formulae, which can be included as snacks or recovery snacks (these should contain more carbohydrate than protein), carbohydrate powders (such as glucose polymers), skim milk powder, sports bars, drinks and gels.

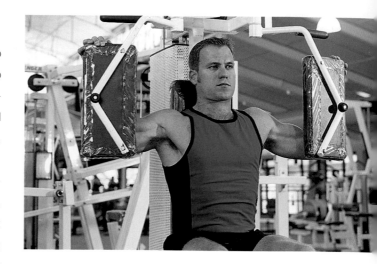

Above right *Body builders are frequently targeted by manufacturers of supplements.*

CAN SUPPLEMENTS CAUSE A POSITIVE DOPING RESULT?

Since the industry is poorly regulated, many popular supplements contain banned ingredients not clearly listed on the label, and the product can be contaminated. Even small amounts of a contaminant (0.02% nandrolone, for instance) can cause a positive test.

Any of the following ingredients, banned by WADA and the International Olympic Committee (IOC), can be found in supplements:

Amphetamines

Ephedrine/ma huang/nor-pseudoephedrine

Strychnine

Pro-hormones:

> Dehydroepiandrosterone (DHEA)

> Androstenedione, androstenediol

> 19-norandrostenedione

> 19-norandrostenediol

The FDA intends to ban the sale of supplements containing ephedrine alkaloids, but some athletes will have old stock (fat burners, for example) that still contain ephedrine.

The controlling bodies put the onus on the athlete to avoid banned substances. Athletes are warned that they are 'responsible for all or any substance detected in samples given by them'.

EVALUATION OF POPULAR SUPPLEMENTS

In this section sports supplements are critically evaluated against the manufacturer's claims. Few supplements have sufficient evidence to support their use.

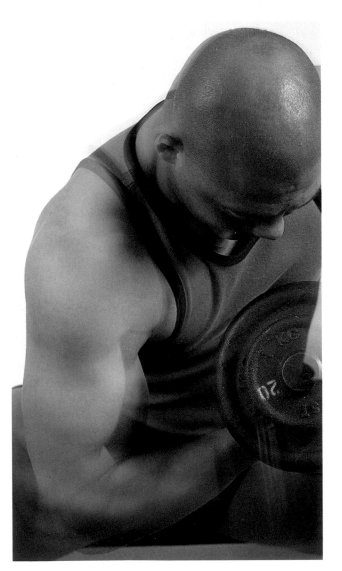

INCREASED MUSCLE MASS
CREATINE

Creatine (methylguanidine acetic acid) is one of the most popular supplements, usually taken in the form of creatine monohydrate. It is an amino acid compound (protein) which occurs naturally in the body (total 120g), 95% of it in muscle (⅔ as phospho creatine and ⅓ as free creatine).

Creatine is not a drug. It is not on the List of Prohibited Substances and Methods of WADA and the IOC, nor is it an illegal substance in terms of the law. It is readily available in supermarkets, pharmacies and health food stores.

Creatine is found in many foods, mostly in meat, fish and other animal products. A person consumes an average of 1–2g of creatine daily; vegetarians much less. Individuals with initial low creatine levels appear to respond much better to creatine supplementation.

WHAT ARE THE EFFECTS OF CREATINE?

Creatine phosphate is involved in a number of functions in exercising muscle. It provides a limited, but rapidly available source of fuel to regenerate ATP (*see the conversion of food to fuel p27*), which is the most important fuel source in the performance of all-out sprints of 5–10 seconds. Maintenance of ATP during anaerobic exercise is dependant on the breakdown of phospho creatine (PCr), freeing the phosphate to bond with adenosine diphosphate (ADP) to form adenosine triphosphate (ATP).

When muscle contracts, ATP is broken down to ADP, catalyzed by the enzyme creatine phosphokinase (CPK). ATP is restored when the CPK reaction is reversed so that the phosphate from phospho creatine (PCr) is again transferred to ADP to form ATP, and creatine is released. It is expressed as:

$$PCr + ADP + H^+ \text{ ion} \leftarrow CPK \rightarrow Cr + ATP$$

Above *Athletes are warned by WADA that they are responsible for everything they ingest and therefore for any banned substance detected in samples given by them, regardless of how the substance got there.*

INCREASED MUSCLE MASS

SUFFICIENT EVIDENCE	INSUFFICIENT OR NO EVIDENCE	COMMENTS AND TIPS
Protein (e.g. whey powders)	Individual amino acids (e.g. arginine ornithine)	Excessive protein intakes can result in fat gain and will not have a further ergogenic effect.
Creatine		Weight gain initially due to water retention and later protein synthesis. (See below for side effects.)
HMB (ß-hydroxy-ß-methylbutyrate)		1.5–3g per day in the early stages of training may reduce muscle damage, decrease body fat and increase muscle mass. May have an additive effect on body composition when combined with creatine. No acute recognized side effects; results from long-term studies still needed.
Carbohydrate + protein	Carbohydrate + wheat hydrolysate + added leucine and phenylalanine	After exercise, ingesting 0.8–1.2g carbohydrate/kg + 0.4g protein/kg has been shown to aid recovery and have anabolic effects.
	BCAA	

Creatine also buffers the hydrogen ions produced within the muscle cells and transports the ATP to that part of the cell that causes muscle contraction.

The effects of creatine include increased power and strength and increased muscle mass, giving a distinct advantage in sports that involve resistance training, repeated bouts of high-intensity sprints (football and tennis) separated by short rest periods (interval sessions of running, cycling and swimming).

By decreasing the recovery time between repeated bouts of exercise, creatine allows the athlete to train more intensely and for a longer period of time, hence becoming bigger and stronger. Creatine can, however, be disadvantageous in endurance sports such as marathon running and long distance cycling because of the increased muscle bulk, affecting the power-to-weight ratio.

WHAT ARE THE SIDE EFFECTS?

There is no scientific evidence of major health risks associated with short-term creatine supplementation. There is anecdotal evidence of high blood pressure, kidney damage and muscle cramps. The safety profile of its long-term use still needs to be established. However, creatine supplementation should be avoided by athletes with impaired kidney function and/or elevated blood pressure.

Its use by children is of growing concern because of the potential damage that can occur to growth plates and the imbalance that will exist with the increase in muscle mass and muscle strength.

Opposite *Creatine supplementation without an appropriate training and dietary regime will not help build muscle.*

GENERAL ADVICE TO ATHLETES

- Previously a rapid loading of 20–25g creatine per day (for 5–7 days) followed by a maintenance dose of 5g per day was recommended, since in most people this increases the creatine stores in the muscle by 10–30%. However, it has been shown that a slow loading of 3g per day will achieve the same increase in a given time (not much more than in a meat eater's diet). Any extra creatine is excreted via the urine.
- Note that creatine + 50–100g carbohydrate (not fructose) maximizes absorption, whereas caffeine impairs absorption. Creatine should be dissolved in adequate fluid and taken after exercise.
- There are 'responders' and 'non-responders' – not all individuals taking creatine show improved performance. It may only be of benefit in specific sports (*see p98*).
- Weight gain within the first few days is probably as a result of water retention.
- Creatine without an appropriate training and dietary regime will have no effect at all on muscle building.
- Creatine should be avoided if there is thermal stress.

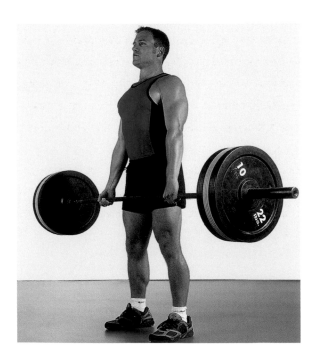

BRANCHED CHAIN AMINO ACIDS (BCAA) – ITS EARLIER HYPOTHESIS WITH CENTRAL FATIGUE

Branched Chain Amino Acids consist of three essential amino acids – leucine, isoleucine and valine. Manufacturers claim better absorption of BCAAs compared to whole (intact) protein found in everyday foods. Unlike the anabolic effects claimed for other individual amino acids, the interest in BCAA in the 1980s related to its role in delaying fatigue. Two mechanisms have been suggested to explain the role of BCAA in delaying fatigue.

The first theory is that BCAA competes with another amino acid, tryptophan, for transport across the blood-brain barrier, so that less tryptophan is converted into serotonin (a chemical associated with drowsiness and central or brain fatigue as opposed to muscle fatigue or fuel depletion).

The other theory is based on the fact that as muscle glycogen levels decrease during prolonged exercise, there is an increased oxidation of fat and BCAA as fuel. Therefore free fatty acid (FFA) levels in the blood start to go up, while the availability of BCAA in the blood decreases. The increase in FFA levels in the blood is accompanied by a release of tryptophan from its binding protein (albumin), thus increasing the level of free tryptophan in the blood. Increased levels of tryptophan in the brain promote the formation of serotonin (which is associated with tiredness). By taking BCAA you can reduce the levels of FFA, which reduces the release of tryptophan from albumin and therefore you have less tryptophan in the blood to promote the formation of serotonin.

Not enough is known to make practical recommendations. Moreover, taking BCAA during exercise may cause ammonia to be produced and this may cause fatigue. Carbohydrate intake during exercise, on the other hand, can not only prevent central fatigue by decreasing free fatty acid levels, but it has the additional benefit of supplying fuel!

More recently the interest in BCAA has shifted to its anabolic effects on muscle mass when taken after exercise.

DECREASED FAT MASS

CAFFEINE

Individuals respond differently to caffeine, but performance-enhancing effects are found at doses as low as 1–3mg/kg of body weight (50–100mg caffeine). There is no additional benefit in taking larger doses and at higher levels you can experience side effects such as nervousness, anxiety, palpitations, headaches and dehydration. The ergogenic effect of caffeine can be due to multiple effects. Several mechanisms have been proposed, including a direct stimulatory effect on the central nervous system (decreased fatigue and increased metabolic rate) to change the perception of effort and increase fatty acid mobilization, thus sparing muscle glycogen. Even though caffeine has been removed from the WADA/IOC list of banned substances, it is still good to be aware of the caffeine content of foods, beverages (energy drinks, sports drinks, tea and coffee), sports gels and drugs to avoid unwanted side effects (*see p67*).

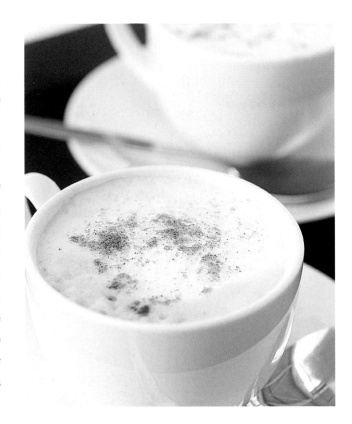

DECREASED FAT MASS

SUFFICIENT EVIDENCE	INSUFFICIENT OR NO EVIDENCE	COMMENTS AND TIPS
Meal replacement formulae		Weight loss results from decreased calorie and fat intake; caution against over-reliance; no variety, limited fibre
	Fat burners such as CLA (conjugated linoleic acid), l-carnitine, pyruvate and chromium picolinate Fat-trappers (chitosan)	
Stimulants and appetite suppressants (ephedrine, ma huang, nor-pseudoephedrine, guarana, caffeine) sometimes used as a stack		Some may cause fat loss in the short term but many of these stimulants (exception caffeine, synephrine and guarana) are banned and have major side effects. NB: Read labels carefully for pseudonyms (e.g. Chinese ephedra and sida cordifolio) used for ephedrine. Note also that many herbals contain other banned substances

INCREASED CARBOHYDRATE STORAGE [CARBO-LOADING]

SUFFICIENT EVIDENCE	INSUFFICIENT OR NO EVIDENCE	COMMENTS AND TIPS
High-carbohydrate supplements (sports drinks, bars, glucose, glucose polymer powders – flavoured and unflavoured)		Sports drinks with a higher concentration of carbohydrate can be used (10–15%). Unflavoured glucose polymer powders can be added to foods and drinks. Powders can be mixed to desired concentration. Bars are compact and are low in fibre. Check products for 'hidden' ingredients e.g. caffeine/guarana/Medium Chain Triglycerides (MCTs).

INCREASED CARBOHYDRATE AVAILABILITY DURING TRAINING/EVENTS

SUFFICIENT EVIDENCE	INSUFFICIENT OR NO EVIDENCE	COMMENTS AND TIPS
High-carbohydrate supplements (sports drinks, bars, gels, glucose, glucose polymer powders)		Appropriate concentration is important to ensure carbohydrate and fluid delivery and to minimize gastrointestinal side effects. Gels are useful when fluid requirements are low and/or when impractical to eat food. Powders can be mixed to desired concentration. Bars are compact and are low in fibre. Check products for 'hidden' ingredients e.g. caffeine/guarana/MCTs.

INCREASED ATP AND CREATINE PHOSPHATE LEVELS

SUFFICIENT EVIDENCE	INSUFFICIENT OR NO EVIDENCE	COMMENTS AND TIPS
Creatine		Some athletes participating in resistance training or repeated bouts of high-intensity sprints separated by short rest periods may benefit.
	ATP Ribose CoQ10	

INCREASED FAT OXIDATION DURING EXERCISE TO SPARE MUSCLE GLYCOGEN

SUFFICIENT EVIDENCE	INSUFFICIENT OR NO EVIDENCE	COMMENTS AND TIPS
	Hydroxy Citric Acid (HCA) l-carnitine MCTs Caffeine	A fat-loading regime may benefit certain athletes (*see pp18, 30, 166–167, 175–176*)

IMPROVED RECOVERY

SUFFICIENT EVIDENCE	INSUFFICIENT OR NO EVIDENCE	COMMENTS AND TIPS
High GI carbohydrate, either on its own or mixed with protein and added electrolytes (e.g. formulae providing 60–70g carbohydrate, 10–30g protein, electrolytes)		Recovery formulae (to be consumed within 30–60 minutes after exercise) are convenient, especially when lacking appetite
	Glutamine	

HYDRATION

SUFFICIENT EVIDENCE	INSUFFICIENT OR NO EVIDENCE	COMMENTS AND TIPS
Sports drinks with 30–70g CHO/litre (15–35g CHO/pt) and sodium		Choose according to event (type and duration) and personal preference (see fluid chapter)

IMPROVED COGNITIVE FUNCTION; IMPROVED REACTION TIMES

SUFFICIENT EVIDENCE	INSUFFICIENT OR NO EVIDENCE	COMMENTS AND TIPS
Caffeine *caffeine can also be ergolytic (worsen performance)		The ability of caffeine to increase alertness can help in prolonged events (*see also p100*)
	Tryptophan BCAA Choline Lecithin Gamma-aminobutyric amino acid Tyrosine	

PREVENTION OF ACID BUILD-UP DURING EXERCISE, AND CRAMPS

BICARBONATE, LACTATE AND CITRATE

Soda-loading is not a banned practice in athletes, but it is not permitted in dogs and horses. Athletes have used soda-loading (or bicarbonate-loading) for over 70 years in an attempt to buffer the acids (hydrogen ions) released during high-intensity exercise and thus to delay the onset of muscle fatigue. Athletes usually ingest about 0.3g sodium bicarbonate (4–5tsp bicarbonate of soda), 0.3–0.5g sodium citrate, or 0.4g sodium lactate per kilogram of body weight 1–2 hours before exercise. There are no foods that produce this effect. Bicarbonate- or citrate-loading may benefit some athletes in events demanding near maximal intensity and lasting 1–7 minutes (400–1500m running, 100–400m swimming, rowing, kayaking events). There is unconfirmed evidence that it may be useful in 30km (19-mile) cycle races. Before trying soda-loading you will need to determine if you are a 'responder' or 'non-responder' (experiment in training). Be aware that these agents can have laxative and other side effects.

PREVENTION OF ACID BUILD-UP DURING EXERCISE, AND CRAMPS

SUFFICIENT EVIDENCE	INSUFFICIENT OR NO EVIDENCE	COMMENTS AND TIPS
Sodium bicarbonate-, lactate-, or citrate-loading		The effectiveness as a buffer and side effects will vary according to the type of compound used.
	Magnesium Zinc Ribose Vitamin E Beta-carotene	Low magnesium levels are not associated with muscle cramps. Other factors like muscle fatigue are more important.

BONE AND JOINT REPAIR AND RECOVERY FROM INJURY

SUFFICIENT EVIDENCE	INSUFFICIENT OR NO EVIDENCE	COMMENTS AND TIPS
Glucosamine sulphate and chondroitin sulphate		Repairs articular cartilage and has mild anti-inflammatory properties. No evidence of benefit in athletes without cartilage damage. Long-term effects are still unknown.
	Proline, lysine, phyto-oestrogens, vitamin K	

OTHER

COLOSTRUM

Colostrum is the milk produced by mammals (human and bovine) within the first 48 hours after birth, before milk is produced. It is rich in all nutrients and also contains antibacterial, hormonal and growth factors. There is no doubt that colostrum is anabolic and of immune benefit to babies, but whether it has similar effects in athletes remains uncertain. It is yet to be determined how much can actually be digested or absorbed by adults.

PROHORMONES – DESIGNER SUPPLEMENTS

Recently there has been a surge in the number of new, unregulated designer sports supplements on the market with awesome claims. Many of these products (either overtly or inadvertently) contain prohormones that can be grouped into testosterone precursors and nandrolone precursors. It is interesting that the findings of various studies published in recent literature reviews showed no support for the claims made by manufacturers. The side effects of these substances, however, cannot be ignored (see below).

Below *Some of the 'magic' claims made for new-age supplements.*

TESTOSTERONE PRECURSORS (PROHORMONES)

Testosterone precursor hormones (e.g. dehydroepiandrosterone (DHEA); androstenedione; androstenediol) provide the necessary materials to increase the production of testosterone in the body. The ingestion of these precursor hormones may result in a positive doping test – if the testosterone to epitestosterone (T:E) ratio is more than 6:1, this constitutes a positive test. If testosterone prohormones are ingested inadvertently, the T:E ratio may remain elevated for up to 24 hours.

The effect of tribulus terrestris, herbal testosterone supplements, zinc magnesium antioxidant (ZMA), and ecdysterone (suma) on drug testing results is unknown.

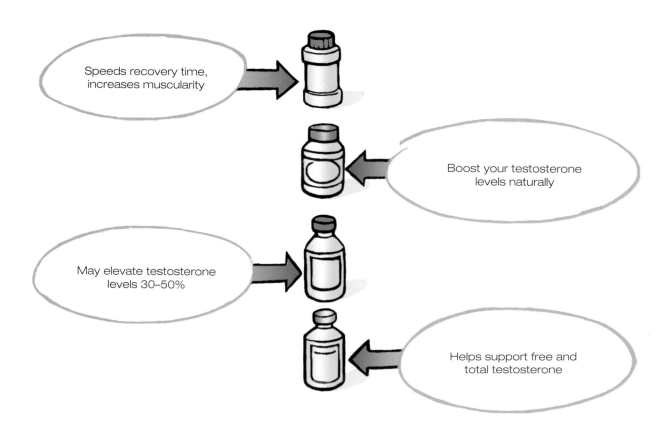

Speeds recovery time, increases muscularity

Boost your testosterone levels naturally

May elevate testosterone levels 30–50%

Helps support free and total testosterone

NANDROLONE PRECURSORS

Nandrolone precursor steroids (i.e. 19-norandrostenedione; 19-norandrostenediol) may increase the production of nandrolone in the body. They may be found in small amounts in other commonly used supplements. If a nandrolone precursor steroid is ingested, it can be converted to nandrolone by the body. The nandrolone is broken down to 19-norandrosterone, which can be found in the urine. The athlete will have a positive drug test if the concentration is greater than 2ng per millilitre. The urine can remain positive for 7–10 days.

Negative side effects of prohormone steroids in general are water retention, hypertension, decreased HDL cholesterol, abnormal liver function tests, mood and behavioural changes and acne.

In males specifically the side effects include impotence and sterility, development of breast tissue, premature baldness and abnormalities of the reproductive system (atrophy of the testes, decreased sperm count, enlargement and cancer of the prostate).

In females the side effects include increased facial and body hair, deepening of the voice, abnormalities of the reproductive system and sexual organs, clitoral enlargement and menstrual problems.

In adolescents steroid use may stunt growth due to the premature closing of growth centres of the bone.

CHECKLIST APPRAISAL

To help you sort reliable information from the questionable, especially when trying to make sense of product claims, you can make use of the adjacent checklist. If products have been on the market for a while, be aware that updated information may not be reflected – for example, there may now be side effects or interactions not previously known. The Internet is also an easy vehicle for spreading myths, hoaxes and rumours.

EVALUATING PRODUCTS AND CLAIMS

SCIENTIFIC VALIDITY

1. Does the amount and form of the active ingredient claimed to be present in the supplement match that used in scientific studies on this ergogenic aid?
2. Does the claim by the manufacturer match the science of nutrition and exercise?
3. Does the ergogenic claim make sense for the sport for which the claim is made?

QUALITY OF SUPPORTIVE EVIDENCE

1. What evidence is provided (scientific or testimonial)?
2. What is the quality of the science? Reputation of the researcher(s)? Journal in which the science is published? Was the research sponsored by a supplement company? Was it a hypothesis-driven, randomized, placebo-controlled, blinded research trial? On humans or in test tubes?
3. Were methods clearly presented so study results could be reproduced?
4. Are results clearly presented in an unbiased manner, with appropriate statistical analysis? Are results feasible, and the conclusions that follow reasonable and based on the data?

SAFETY AND LEGALITY OF THE ERGOGENIC AID

1. Is the product safe? Will it compromise the health of an individual? Does the product contain some toxic or unknown substance? Is the product contraindicated in people with a particular health problem?
2. Will the use of the product preclude other factors in optimizing performance (training, for example)?
3. Is the product illegal or banned by any athletic or sporting organization? Is there a legal limit to the use of the ergogenic aid, in terms of dose?

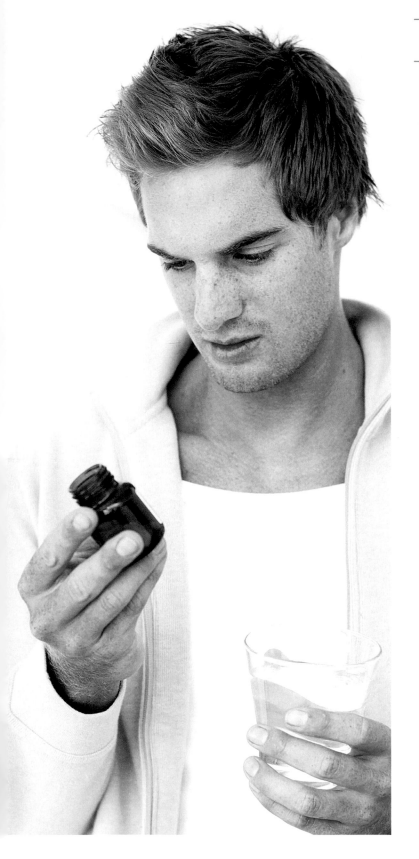

Additional tips and recommendations

1. Supplements should only be taken when there is proof that the diet cannot provide the quantities of nutrients needed. This requires a thorough assessment by a registered sports dietitian/nutritionist.

2. Dosages of supplements need to be calculated to avoid overdose. Avoid taking a variety of supplements supplying the same nutrients (polypharmacy) and note that more is not always better since there is an optimal level of nutrient functioning beyond which they become detrimental (*see p107*). Excessive intakes of individual nutrients (vitamin A, for example) can either be toxic or teratogenic (lead to birth defects) and others may prevent the absorption of essential nutrients (for instance, a high calcium intake inhibits iron absorption). The form of the supplement may determine its bioavailability. For example, amino acid supplements in the L-form are better utilized than those in D-form.

3. Individuals may respond differently. Try and test diet and supplement well before competition.

4. Supplements required in clinical situations require a medical diagnosis and should only be prescribed by a sports physician or dietitian in writing.

   NOTE: Athletes should check with their sporting federation about its supplement policy. Athletes should request written prescriptions for supplements and obtain a quality control certificate from the manufacturer (this should demonstrate that the product batch has been tested at an independent IOC-accredited laboratory and has been shown to be free of prohibited substances) as well as legally binding documentation listing all the different products they produce and that the company accepts full liability for a positive doping test as a result of the use thereof.

5. No persons under the age of 18 should take any sport-specific supplements without advice from a sports physician or dietitian.

6. All supplement labels should be carefully studied and ingredients noted. Look for hidden relationships between ingredients, unstated ingredients and avoid banned pro-hormone supplements. Note that the term 'natural' does not mean that a product is healthful and safer to use than drugs. Many weight-loss products claim to be 'natural' or 'herbal' but their ingredients may interact with drugs or may be dangerous for people with certain medical conditions. Note that dietary supplement manufacturers may not necessarily include warnings about potential adverse effects on the labels of their products.

7. Even if the product says 'IOC permitted' this does not mean it is safe to use. The IOC does not endorse any nutritional supplements.

NOTE: You can obtain more information on how the FDA regulates dietary supplements and on the manufacturers' responsibilities for the products they market at Questions and Answers http://www.cfsan.fda.gov/~dms/ds-faq.html For more information on the anti-doping code, see www.wada-ama.org

8. See also Food Standards Agency: www.food.gov.uk

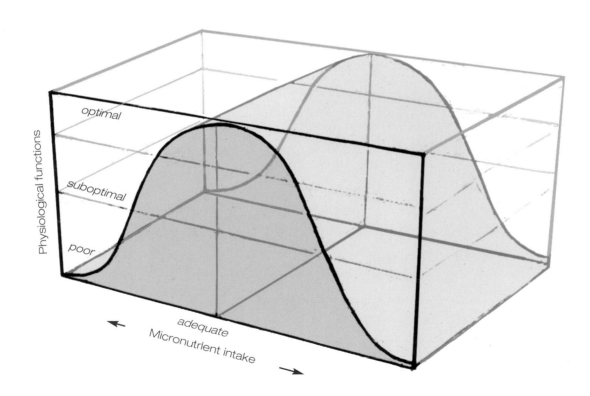

Above *Optimal micronutrient intake falls within a range and performance is not enhanced after the minimum requirements are met.*

Opposite *Read labels carefully to check for hidden ingredients and false claims.*

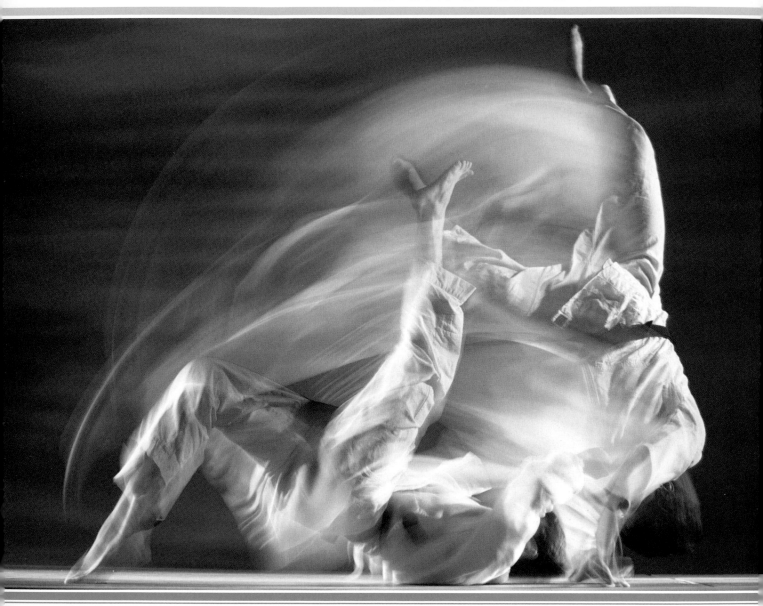

chapter 8

WEIGHT-MAKING SPORTS

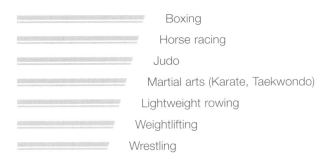

Boxing

Horse racing

Judo

Martial arts (Karate, Taekwondo)

Lightweight rowing

Weightlifting

Wrestling

'I remember feeling that I had just won a victory by making the weight for a match and then I realized that I still had to wrestle' – Lefavi, cited in *Sports Under Fire*, by Bednar C. 1998

Weight-making sports impose specific weight limits for competition in order to match opponents of equal weight and ability. For example, a 72kg (159 lb) middle-weight boxer will be more competitive if he can drop a few kilograms to compete in the lower weight division of under 68kg (150 lb), rather than fight against much heavier opponents. As a result, many athletes participating in weight-making sports employ tactics to downsize just before an event.

A low body fat level is a distinct advantage in weight-category sports, because it improves the power-to-weight ratio and also helps increase an athlete's rate of acceleration. Due to the weight-making pressures of the sport and the possibility of being disqualified before a competition, many athletes develop unhealthy eating and drinking patterns, which include weight cycling (yo-yo dieting) and binge eating. These practices not only have a negative effect on performance, but also carry other risks, both physiological and psychological, such as mood swings.

Making weight need not be a problem, provided strategies are implemented in good time, rather than hours before competition. This is contrary to the common belief that drastic weight loss is an essential part of the sporting culture. Weight-loss techniques commonly used by athletes to make weight are:

- drastic dehydration
- spitting
- forced nosebleeds
- food and fluid restriction
- increased exercise
- fasting
- sauna
- rubber suits
- laxatives
- vomiting
- use of banned substances.

PHYSICAL DEMANDS AND CHARACTERISTICS

Although the competitive event might be of short duration, training usually involves long hours of high-intensity training with high-energy demands. Training taxes all the energy systems (*see pp28, 148*) used during competition and also incorporates skill and technique. For example, male and female rowers can expend as much as 25,000–29,000kJ (5950–6900kcal) and 21,000–25,000kJ (5000–5950kcal) per day respectively, yet these athletes often report consuming low-energy diets. It is therefore believed that these athletes become energy efficient; they are able to train and compete on far fewer calories than expected. This energy efficiency makes weight loss more difficult so that athletes resort to more and more drastic measures. Weight fluctuations and changes in diet and activity also alter metabolism, endocrine function and body composition.

Opposite top *Jockeys have to weigh in before and directly after each race in which they compete.*
Opposite bottom *Severely restricted energy intakes and rapid weight loss will affect the athlete's ability to concentrate.*

BOXING
AMATEUR

COMPETITION AND WEIGH-IN PROCEDURES

Each bout consists of four two-minute rounds (maximum five) with a minute rest in-between. Between rounds boxers can receive fluid and coaching advice.

Competitors box every second day and may be expected to box four to five times during the tournament. The main objective is to score maximum points.

All competitors weigh in on the first day of competition between 08:00 and 10:00. On following days only those who are drawn to box are expected to weigh in, again between 08:00 and 10:00. There should be at least a three-hour gap between weighing-in and competing.

AMATEUR WEIGHT CATEGORIES

MALE	DIVISION
Less than 48kg (106 lb)	Light fly weight
48–51kg (106–112 lb)	Fly weight
51–54kg (112–119 lb)	Bantam weight
54–57kg (119–125 lb)	Feather weight
57–60kg (125–132 lb)	Light weight
60–63.5kg (132–140 lb)	Light welter weight
63.5–67kg (140–147 lb)	Welter weight
67–71kg (147–156 lb)	Light middle weight
71–75kg (156–165 lb)	Middle weight
75–81kg (165–178 lb)	Light heavy weight
81–91kg (178–200 lb)	Heavy weight
91kg (200 lb) and over	Super heavy

For female boxers the weight categories range from 45kg (99 lb) to over 81kg (178 lb).

BOXING
PROFESSIONAL
COMPETITION AND WEIGH-IN PROCEDURES

World title fights are fought over 12 three-minute rounds. The number of rounds per fight varies between 4 and 12 (with a maximum of 15). Competitors usually fight three to four times per year. The main objective is to score a knock-out.

In Australia competitors weigh in anywhere up to half an hour before a fight, but 8–10 hours before a title fight. Competitors in any of the world boxing organizations' title bouts weigh in 24 hours prior to a fight.

Weight divisions may vary slightly between countries and boxing associations.

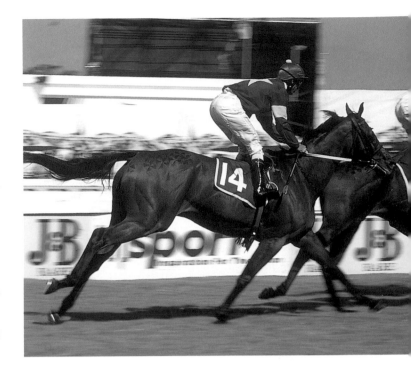

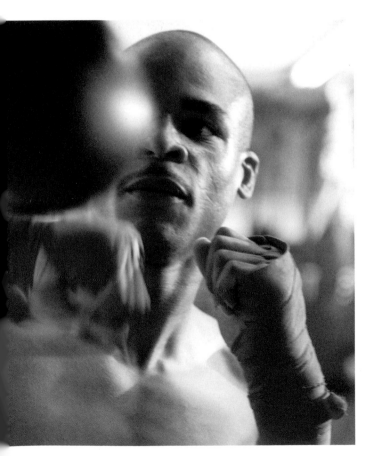

HORSE RACING – JOCKEYS
COMPETITION AND WEIGH-IN PROCEDURES

Races are conducted over various distances, usually 1000–2000m (1094–2188yd) lasting 1–2 minutes, but can be as long as 3200m (3500yd). Jockeys can have up to eight rides during one racing session, which lasts roughly 5–6 hours.

All jockeys weigh in 30 to 45 minutes before each race in which they compete, and again directly after the race.

WEIGHT CATEGORIES

Minimum weight for any race varies between races and between countries, and horses are weight-handicapped according to ability or age. According to Australian Rules no horse shall have its weight burden reduced below 43.5kg (96 lb), including saddle and accessories, and the minimum weight to be carried by any horse in a handicap flat race shall not be less than 46kg (101 lb). If a horse carries less or more than the weight it should carry, it may be disqualified for the race and the jockey will be fined.

JUDO

COMPETITION AND WEIGH-IN PROCEDURES

Each bout lasts four minutes for females and five minutes for males. The competition lasts one day only. A competitor can expect to contest four to five (up to eight) bouts during the competition. A minimum of 10 minutes must elapse between bouts. The aim is to throw or pin an opponent in a ground hold.

Weigh-in starts at least two hours before the scheduled start of the competition. Weight can be checked unofficially (trial) until the official weigh–in period one hour before competition.

KARATE

COMPETITION AND WEIGH-IN PROCEDURES

There are team events, but these have no weight categories. The individual bouts last three minutes for males and two minutes for females. Depending on the number of competitors in the tournament, competitors will fight six to eight times. Competition for a weight category is completed over one day.

At international level, weigh-in is usually conducted the day before the tournament starts, but is in the discretion of the organizing committee.

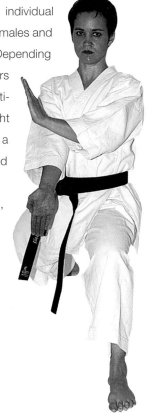

WEIGHT CATEGORIES

MALE	FEMALE
Less than 60kg (132 lb)	Less than 48kg (106 lb)
66kg (145 lb)	52kg (114 lb)
73kg (161 lb)	57kg (125 lb)
81kg (178 lb)	63kg (139 lb)
90kg (198 lb)	70kg (154 lb)
100kg (220 lb)	78kg (172 lb)
More than 100kg (220 lb)	Above 78kg (172 lb)

WEIGHT CATEGORIES

MALE	FEMALE
Below 60kg (132.3 lb)	< 53kg (116.87 lb)
60.01–65kg (132.32–143.32 lb)	53.01–60kg (116.89–132.3 lb)
65.01–70kg (143.34–154.35 lb)	60.01kg (132.32 lb) and above
70.01–75kg (154.37–165.38 lb)	
75.01–80kg (165.4–176.4 lb)	
80.01kg (176.42 lb) and above	

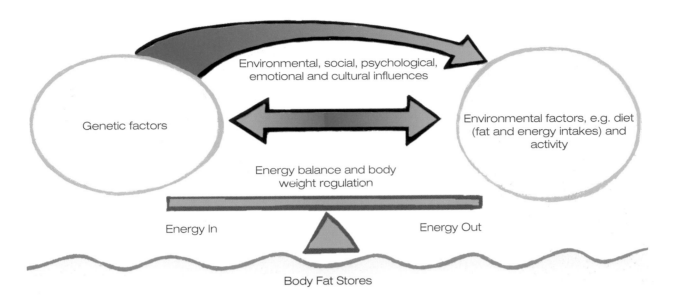

Body Fat Stores

METHODS USED FOR FAT LOSS

Athletes often use extreme measures to manipulate body weight or fat to improve performance and appearance.

The most effective approach is to combine energy restriction (diet) with energy expenditure (exercise). Exercise, besides burning calories, has the additional benefits of increasing muscle mass, increasing the resting metabolic rate and thermic effects of food (TEF). It also has 'feel-good' benefits, which helps to motivate dietary compliance.

FAD DIETS

Unscientific dietary regimes appeal because they promise quick weight loss, but their use may also result in fatigue and decreased performance.

The popular diets represented on the continuum below have manipulated the macronutrient composition (protein, carbohydrate and fat) on the premise that one or other macronutrient dramatically affects weight loss. Unfortunately for most, there is little scientific evidence to support their approach.

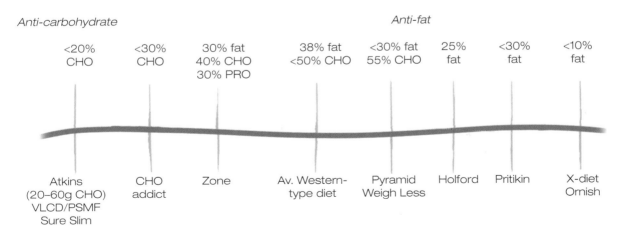

CHO = carbohydrate; VLCD = very low calorie diet; PSMF = protein-sparing modified fast.
Percentages given are of total energy intake.

HIGH-PROTEIN/LOW-CARBOHYDRATE [OR ATKINS AND SUGAR BUSTERS]

CLAIM

'Low-fat diets don't work; sugar and refined carbohydrates are the real culprits because they cause an excessive insulin response. This may result in fat storage and low blood sugar levels causing hunger.'

The Atkins diet does not restrict protein, fat or calories in the belief that the combination of protein and fat promotes satiety resulting in individuals eating less and thus losing weight. Protagonists of the diet claim that fat will also be broken down by the body (because of the low carbohydrate content), resulting in the formation of ketones (ketosis).

FACT

Ketosis is never a desirable state. Ketogenic diets, regardless of the level of energy intake, bring about significant metabolic changes and the diuretic effect of ketosis may affect kidney function through fluid and electrolyte losses. Ketosis might cause nausea, light-headedness and fatigue. The Atkins diet is also high in total and saturated fat, which may over time increase the risk of heart disease and some cancers. There is also evidence that more total energy is consumed on high-fat diets. Although weight may be lost initially, long-term studies are needed to assess efficacy. The minimal carbohydrate intake does not allow individuals to consume the fibre and phytonutrients found in fruit, vegetables and whole grains. Low-carbohydrate diets do not support the regular physical activity needed for sustained weight loss.

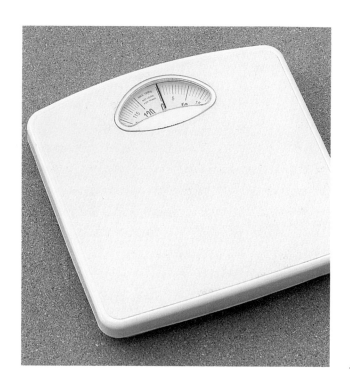

FAT-FREE/HIGH-CARBOHYDRATE [X-DIET, DEAN ORNISH]

CLAIM

'Fat is the enemy and the cause of many health problems.'

The 'X-diet' only includes foods containing less than 3g fat per 100g (3⅓ oz), but allows sugar and other carbohydrates in unlimited quantities, whereas Dean Ornish promotes a 10% fat diet focusing on whole foods, fruit, vegetables, grains, beans and soya products (essentially vegetarian).

FACT

Fat has essential functions and cannot be excluded (in fact, the X-diet advises supplementation with essential fatty acids). Unlimited carbohydrate intake also provides additional energy. Controlled studies support the long-standing evidence that energy intake is a primary factor in weight gain. Fat-free diets are highly restrictive and difficult to maintain.

The Dean Ornish programme, however, encourages a total lifestyle change and is not meant to be a quick fix.

Above right *Weight measured on a scale is not an accurate indication of body fat levels.*

MODERATE-TO-LOW CARBOHYDRATE [THE ZONE]

CLAIM

'The Zone is a metabolic state that can be reached by everyone and maintained indefinitely on a lifelong basis.'

The founder of the Zone diet, Barry Sears, believes that carbohydrates are the reason why people are fat. He promotes carbohydrates with a low glycaemic index (GI) in favour of high GI foods. High-carbohydrate diets increase blood insulin levels (insulin is a hormone that regulates glucose), resulting in an accumulation of body fat.

FACT

There is some truth in the fact that insulin promotes fat storage, but this is generally well regulated unless you are insulin resistant. Although different carbohydrates elicit different insulin responses, the practical application is quite complicated as most people enjoy mixed meals.

Carbohydrate is not the only culprit, but excessive energy intake in general will lead to obesity. The Zone diet recommends a composition of 40% carbohydrate, 30% protein and 30% fat for every meal. Since this is often not practical, you need specific Zone-endorsed products. Remember, protein often contains hidden fat, and fat supplies more than double the energy compared to carbohydrates.

It seems that the reason for weight loss is due to the limited energy intake as well as the time spent on these complicated calculations. Furthermore, the recommended energy and carbohydrate intakes are insufficient to support the exercise required for weight loss.

RECOGNIZING FAD DIETS

The diet:

- recommends large quantities of a specific food (reliance on a 'miracle food')
- recommends a particular supplement or food replacement
- enforces food combinations and/or requires a very limited energy intake
- excessively restricts carbohydrate-rich foods
- has not been scientifically tested and challenges current scientific thinking
- promises a quick fix
- does not necessarily address the cause of the problem, such as lack of exercise or overeating due to boredom, loneliness or depression.

DIET AIDS

Like fad diets, the use of supplements and/or drugs to assist weight loss is a major temptation for athletes. Despite claims, dietary supplements promoted for weight loss lack scientific support. Furthermore, many of the over-the-counter aids or fat-cutters can contain banned substances and/or have unwanted side effects.

NUTRITION GAME PLAN

Long-term weight maintenance and the prevention of weight cycling can be achieved with simple strategies.

GOAL SETTING AND DIETARY ASSESSMENT

There needs to be consensus about weight-loss goals between coach and athlete and any other member of the management team. The most effective approach is an individualized programme targeting and addressing specific areas that contribute to weight gain. For example, the excessive use of supplements (inappropriate use of high-protein shakes), high-fat fast foods (lack of cooking skills) and snacks, no travel or pre-competition plan (overdoing it at the buffet table) and excessive alcohol consumption (post-game social and peer pressure) are all factors that can make weight management more difficult. The chapter on Making a Plan (*pp44–57*) describes several practical strategies to address common nutritional challenges.

ENERGY INTAKE

The total energy intake recommended should not allow a weight loss of more than 0.5–1kg (1–2 lb) per week. This can be achieved with an energy deficit of 2100kJ (500kcal) per day. Alternatively a body fat loss judged by skinfold measurements (*see p126*), of a maximum of 20mm–40mm per month, is also recommended. Energy intake should not be less than 6300kJ (1500kcal) per day. Athletes who are energy efficient may require fewer calories, but should consult with a sports dietitian.

MACRONUTRIENT INTAKE

Carbohydrate intake should always be sufficient to cover training demands with enough protein to ensure satiety and to prevent loss of lean muscle tissue. Since fat is the most energy-dense nutrient, providing 38kJ or 9kcal per gram (at least 2.5 times more energy per gram than carbohydrate or protein), and hardly has any performance benefits in training, it makes sense to target and reduce fat calories in the diet. The limited amount of fat included in the diet should be rich in polyunsaturated fats since these are more easily oxidized (burned). Alcohol is also a significant source of calories and needs to be reduced.

FAT IN THE DIET MAY MAKE WEIGHT CONTROL MORE CHALLENGING

REASONS TO REDUCE DIETARY FAT

- Fat contains at least two and a half times more energy than starchy foods or animal protein. It is, therefore, easy to ingest excessive energy from fat without necessarily having large portion sizes.
- The body uses the energy from fat very efficiently and fat in the diet can easily be converted to body fat.
- The body can store almost unlimited quantities of dietary fat. By comparison, only small amounts of starchy foods and sugars can be stored in muscle and the liver.
- Fats have a weak effect on the long-term control of appetite and actually have little impact on the feeling of satiety or fullness. This can lead to overeating – see comparison of nutrient properties. Protein, on the other hand, has a positive effect on satiety and, like carbohydrate, also has a low storage capacity in the body and tends to be readily oxidized.

COMPARISON OF NUTRIENT PROPERTIES

CHARACTERISTIC	PROTEIN	CARBOHYDRATE	FAT
Satiety	high	intermediate	low
Hunger suppression	high	high	low
Energy density	low	low	high
Body's capacity to store it	low	low	high

MENU A	SERVING SIZE	ENERGY
HIGH ENERGY DENSITY		
Fettuccine Alfredo	240g (½ lb)	1950kJ (464kcal)
Garlic bread	2 slices	680kJ (162kcal)
Margarine/butter	10ml (2tsp)	378kJ (90kcal)
Fresh vegetable salad	125ml (½ cup)	84kJ (20kcal)
Italian-style dressing	12.5ml (1tbsp)	403kJ (96kcal)
Cheesecake	90g (3 oz)	1063kJ (254kcal)
TOTAL	452g (1 lb)	4560kJ (1086kcal)

MENU B	SERVING SIZE	ENERGY
LOW ENERGY DENSITY		
Spaghetti with tomato-marinara sauce	450g (1 lb)	2030kJ (483kcal)
French bread	3 slices	1020kJ (243kcal)
Fresh vegetable salad	500ml (2 cups)	252kJ (60kcal)
Fat-free dressing/balsamic vinegar	37.5ml (3tbsp)	244kJ (58kcal)
Italian-style vegetables	(1 cup)	310kJ (74kcal)
Fresh strawberries	500ml (2 cups)	378kJ (90kcal)
Sweetened reduced-fat cream	25ml (2tbsp)	328kJ (78kcal)
TOTAL	1279g (3 lb)	4560kJ (1086kcal)

FIBRE INTAKE

Add bulk, especially if you struggle to control appetite, by replacing sports drinks, juice and colddrinks with low-calorie drinks and fruit that provides fibre without additional calories.

MEAL FREQUENCY

Avoid skipping meals. Regular meals ensure constant blood glucose levels and prevent overindulging at later meals.

REGULATE PORTION SIZES

Consider pre-packed meals or meal replacement formulae with predetermined energy values. Familiarize yourself with typical portion sizes.

BE ORGANIZED AND HAVE A PLAN

Take appropriate snacks to training sessions and avoid the temptation to buy high-fat snacks at training venues.

PERIODIZATION

When training is reduced in the off-season or due to injury, energy intake must be adjusted accordingly.

OTHER ESSENTIAL INTERVENTIONS

- **Exercise:** Modify your current training programme to increase your energy expenditure, but take into consideration access to specific facilities, time and the potential for overuse of certain muscle groups resulting in injury.
- **Behaviour modification:** Strategies to help you stick with your weight-loss plan include social support, problem solving and stimulus control (identifying triggers that may lead to overeating, such as boredom or stress).

Left *Two dinner menus of equal energy content that differ dramatically in fat content and total volume.*

CORE COMPONENTS FOR EFFECTIVE WEIGHT-LOSS DIETS

Diets promoting effective weight loss and management should have the following core components:

- The inclusion of a variety of foods that meet your daily nutrient requirements (other than energy). Energy intake should not be less than 5000kJ (1200kcal), or vitamin and mineral shortfalls will occur.
- The ideal daily menu should comprise 50–60% of calories from carbohydrate, about 15–20% from protein and 20–35% from fat.
- The diet should improve overall health without leaving you feeling hungry, faint or fatigued.
- The diet should promote and establish long-term healthy eating patterns.
- The diet should fit in with your tastes, habits and lifestyle.
- Self-monitoring – the use of food diaries – can reinforce healthy eating patterns and help identify those foods or even situations (triggers) that cause you to 'lose control' over your eating.
- The support and involvement of close family and friends should be encouraged.

Body Mass Index

Body Mass Index (BMI) is a measure of body weight relative to height calculated by dividing weight in kilograms by height in metres squared. It can be used to determine if people are overweight or obese and is a better predictor of health risk than weight alone. This formula is accurate for adults other than body builders, competitive athletes, and pregnant or breastfeeding women.

A BMI of 18.5 up to 25 refers to a healthy weight, a BMI of 25 up to 30 refers to overweight and a BMI of 30 or higher refers to obese.

CASE STUDY
FEELING BLOWN UP

BACKGROUND

Ms Flight* was a 19-year-old ballet dancer, sharing a studio apartment with a previously anorexic ballet dancer. Both of them danced at a New York ballet school. Ms Flight was amenorrhic (not menstruating regularly).

She was always 'tiny,' but recalled that at the age of 16 she rapidly gained an 'unusually large' amount of weight (2kg; 4.4 lb!). She was currently the thinnest she had ever been, weighing 47kg (103.6 lb). With a height of 1.59m (5ft 2 in) and body fat content of 20%, she wanted to weigh 43kg (95 lb). The dancing school had threatened to dismiss her if she developed anorex-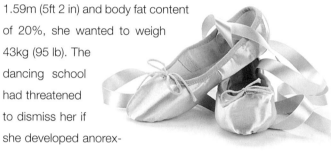
ia nervosa and insisted that she consulted a dietitian.

DIETARY AND TRAINING HISTORY

Ms Flight danced for a total of four hours a day (two hours in the morning and two hours in the evening).

She followed a vegetarian diet, eating the same food every day (*see opposite*). She had eaten no red meat for the previous five years and no chicken for two years. She used to eat fish, but recently cut this out of her diet because 'it made her feel bigger'. She had an aversion to cheese and bananas, but tried to boost her protein intake with milkshakes, which she did not really enjoy. She made a pact not to eat bread and pasta, but loved to eat canned ratatouille and refried beans and, for protein, included three egg whites per week. She allowed herself to succumb to eating two boiled sweets and 10 mints every day. She drank 2–3ℓ (4–6pt) mineral water and diet colddrink every day.

* Name changed to protect client confidentiality.

BREAKFAST

250ml (1 cup) fat-free yoghurt

1 apple

Coffee with skim milk and 10ml (2tsp) sugar

LUNCH

Mixed Chinese free vegetables with a dash of
soya sauce OR a fat-free soup

1 grapefruit

4 rice cakes with apricot jam

SUPPER

2 large bowls of fat-free salad OR soup

A 410g (14 oz) can refried beans OR ratatouille

RECOMMENDATIONS

MAIN CONCERNS

With these restrained eating habits, the highly restricted diet and distorted beliefs about food, Ms Flight was surely developing an eating disorder. The dietitian discussed the implications of reducing her weight even further. This would reduce her body mass index (BMI) from 18.6 to 17, the latter value falling within the category of anorexia nervosa (see p72). Ms Flight was persuaded to maintain her current weight, but to change her body composition by increasing her lean muscle mass while losing body fat. This approach would improve her training, reduce the risk of injury, improve her health and help with long-term weight maintenance.

There were several major dietary concerns (inadequate intakes of energy, carbohydrate, protein, calcium and iron as well as limited variety, food aversions and beliefs) which all needed attention. Priorities were established and an action plan worked out. Ms Flight chose to start with changes that were easily sustainable as this would build up her confidence. She agreed to see the dietitian on a regular basis for ongoing monitoring and support.

DIETARY ADVICE

The dietitian explained the energy contribution from the different macronutrients and their effects on weight. Misconceptions were discussed, which put Ms Flight's mind at ease.

Initial changes, that did not require major food preparation, were recommended.

ENERGY, MACRO- AND MICRONUTRIENTS

- It was decided to keep total energy intake the same, but to include more variety, more nutrients and to change the energy composition to include more protein.
- Sweets, sugar and jam were contributing up to 1050kJ (250kcal) per day. She was advised to swap these for protein, which would also provide her with much-needed iron and calcium. Foods recommended included tofu, fat-free yoghurt, more egg whites, hummus as a spread (at lunch for protein), lentils, peanut butter and fish or sushi.

FIBRE AND FOODS THAT CAUSE BLOATING

The large amounts of fibre consumed, mainly at night, probably contributed to her bloated feeling. By eating less beans or replacing beans with split lentils and rice she would reduce the fibre content and improve the protein quality. Fluid intake seemed excessive and was probably aggravating the discomfort. She was advised to modify and distribute her fibre intake throughout the day, by having wholewheat or rye crackers instead of rice cakes at lunch, for instance.

SUPPLEMENTS

It would be difficult to consume adequate dietary iron on this diet, so it was recommended that her iron status be checked before considering supplementation.

Ms Flight also had her training programme revised to include more resistance work. This, combined with her adjusted diet, helped her to achieve her goal over time, without severe dietary deprivation.

CASE STUDY
SKATING THIN, ON ICE

BACKGROUND

Melissa,* a 14-year-old national figure skater, was constantly tired, lacked appetite and had difficulty in managing her weight, which fluctuated between 53kg (117 lb) and 58kg (128 lb), depending on what diet she was trying out. At the time of her consultation her weight was 53kg (117 lb), height 1.67m (5ft 6 in), body fat mass 20.9%, and a sum of seven skinfolds of 69.4mm (*see p126*). She recently sustained a

stress fracture. Her mother complained that the situation at home had become very tense and that Melissa was 'giving everyone at home a hard time considering all the money they sacrificed to put her through figure skating'. She was also concerned that Melissa was spending a lot of money on weight-loss diets and products, which seemed to change from week to week. She could not understand why Melissa 'could not just eat whatever was put in front of her'.

* Name changed to protect client confidentiality.

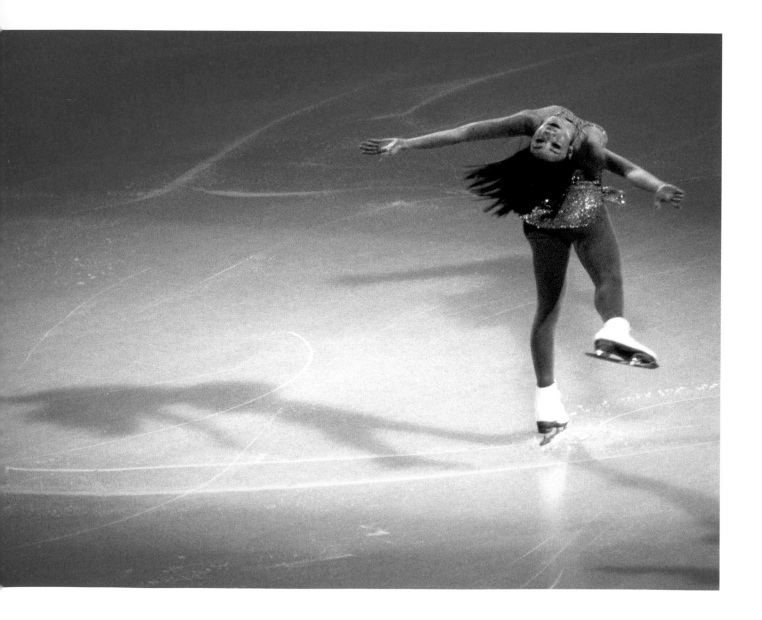

DIETARY AND TRAINING HISTORY

Melissa trained 1½ hours (in the gym or skating) from Monday to Thursday. Friday was a rest day. She skated three hours on Saturday and two hours on Sunday.

Melissa came to her appointment with a food diary describing her food intake over the previous week. Her daily intake was a slight variation of the following:

BREAKFAST
1 medium apple
250ml (1 cup) high-fibre breakfast cereal
160ml (⅔ cup) skim milk
1 cup of coffee

FIRST BREAK
1 banana
2 pitted dates

SECOND BREAK
2 slices brown bread
60g (2 oz) tinned pink salmon
cucumber, carrots, green pepper

15:30 (HOME)
½ slice bread
4 jelly beans

SUPPER
90g (3 oz) chicken breast
spinach, carrots, baby marrow and butternut

EXTRA
8 artificial sweeteners, beetroot

In the six weeks prior to eating this way, she had lost 3kg (6.6 lb) on the Atkins diet (high protein), which she followed for two weeks. She then switched to the Zone diet for the following three weeks and regained the 3kg (6.6 lb) lost. In desperation she resorted to expensive shakes for a week.

RECOMMENDATIONS

MAIN CONCERNS

Following fad diets was creating a pattern of weight cycling and body composition changes. The diets were either expensive, or impractical (did not take the family set-up into consideration). They also did not take her training requirements into account. The diet she was following for the week prior to the consultation was the closest to ideal and was a good basis to work from.

DIETARY ADVICE

Melissa was complimented on her recent efforts and encouraged to continue eating this way. However, her eating plan was fine-tuned to meet her training demands and to allow for long-term weight management. The risks associated with the previous attempts at weight loss were explained to her – that these high-protein, low-carbohydrate, restrictive and very low calorie diets were all contributing to her symptoms of fatigue, the stress fracture, her inability to concentrate and low blood glucose levels.

She was advised to increase energy intake gradually (both carbohydrate and protein with little fat) and to introduce smaller, more frequent, meals and snacks to regulate blood sugar levels. Iron and calcium intakes could be improved by introducing lean meat and fat-free dairy products.

Melissa's mother was included in the consultations to ensure a consistent message and to explain Melissa's specific needs. It was also necessary to get an understanding of the family's typical diet, so that the the family's needs could be incorporated, and Melissa's needs met with minimum modification and disruption.

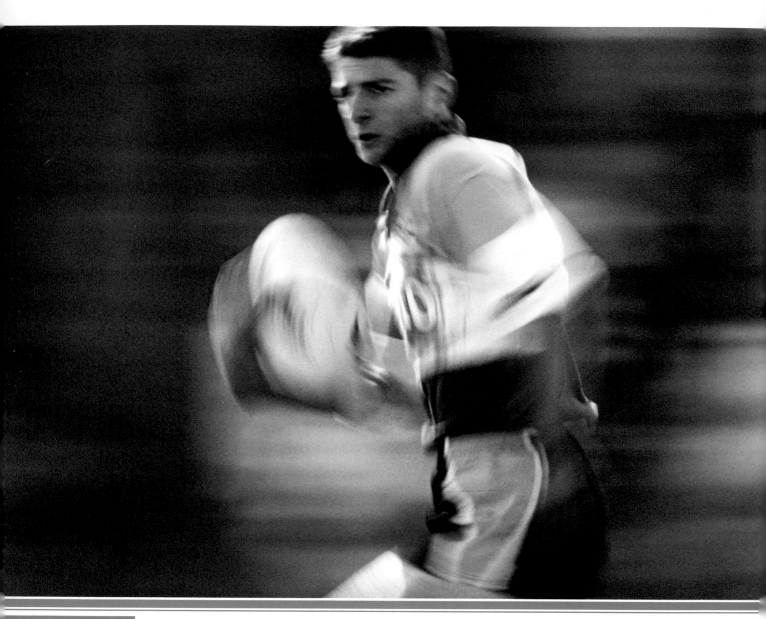

chapter 10

BURSTS OF ENERGY, RAPID RECOVERY

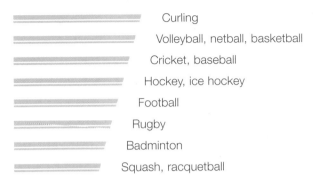

Curling

Volleyball, netball, basketball

Cricket, baseball

Hockey, ice hockey

Football

Rugby

Badminton

Squash, racquetball

'Inside each England rugby player is a real person. It's just that he needs significantly more food than the rest of us.'
– Cook and catering expert Anne Menzies.

Common to all these team and racquet sports is the intermittent, high intensity of play, which places great demands on both the anaerobic and aerobic energy systems (*see pp28, 148*). Players are required to perform at a fast pace, recover quickly and have stamina and endurance, especially when games may be drawn out over time as in tennis. Aerobic fitness assists recovery between bursts of play. Concentration, skill, strategy, agility, explosive strength and sometimes jumping ability are other factors that determine success in these sports.

It has taken some time for nutrition to be recognized as an important performance-enhancing factor in team sports, probably due to the strong culture and tradition of team sports (for instance, supplementation or alcohol consumption may be part of the culture of a specific sport). In comparison to running or cycling, measuring the effect of nutrition on performance in team sports is complicated by the different positions of play, and it would require field-based measurements in different environmental conditions. Although there are only a few studies looking at the role of nutrition in team sports, there is no doubt that a well-organized game plan that involves a holistic approach in a team environment, separate from each individual player's requirements, will enhance performance. A team recovery nutrition plan after training or competition, setting up team rooms, and standardized menus when travelling, are just some of the strategies that can be implemented.

PHYSICAL DEMANDS AND CHARACTERISTICS

Today's team players participate in more games with each passing season, limiting their off-season time. Travel is a huge challenge and they may even be juggling the demands of training and competition with full-time jobs.

Within a team, individual players' requirements will differ according to their position of play. There may also be other differences within the team such as age; cultural; socio-economic; and home circumstances; and lifestyle, which will affect their nutrition requirements.

ENERGY DEMANDS OF THE SPORT

Recent analysis of current field games shows that players cover more distance at a higher intensity with less time for recovery, compared to their counterparts from several years ago. The physiological demands of the game have intensified so that today's players need to be fitter, faster, and stronger.

Training loads will vary according to the time of the season and according to the level of play, but training usually includes general conditioning, weight training, explosive gym work, skill, speed, interval training and team practice. During the season, matches place additional demands on recovery and muscle glycogen stores. An inadequate carbohydrate intake will interfere with both the sprint and endurance components of performance.

> **Above** *A high-energy, high-carbohydrate, high-protein, low-fat diet (and training) is needed to achieve low body fat and high muscle mass.*

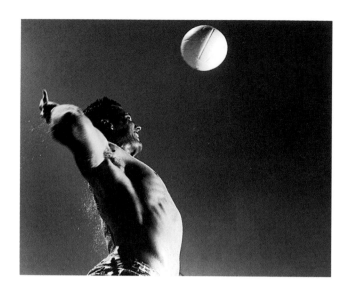

LOW BODY FAT LEVELS AND INCREASED MUSCLE MASS

Different sports have different requirements, as do individual players within the same sport. Typically, players tend to have higher body fat levels at the start of a season. Training and heavy match schedules soon reduce their percentage body fat. Players come in all shapes and sizes, but lower body fat levels are desirable generally as this will maximize speed and agility, and improve heat tolerance and stamina.

Increased muscle mass and power are also required for many of these sports. For example, basketball, football/soccer and rugby players need to be strong and have good body positioning to withstand the contact in a game.

ENVIRONMENT

Many sports evolved in colder climates, but are now played all year, often in hotter climates, thus affecting fluid requirements. External factors such as uniforms, clothing, headgear, gum guards, and whether the sport is played indoors, outdoors, or in water, also affect nutritional needs. Players often mistakenly believe that when playing in a controlled environment, such as an indoor stadium, their performance won't be affected by dehydration, or that it is not necessary to drink when it is cold.

COMMON NUTRITION ISSUES

A single game might not deplete the fuel stores of a trained athlete, but the combination of regular training and competition will have a carry-over effect and slowly deplete reserves.

For week-round recovery, and to prevent progressive fatigue, a habitual high-energy, high-carbohydrate diet is required. Protein needs may be increased to build and maintain muscle mass and for recovery. Fat should always be limited. Immediately after training and competition, specific strategies need to be implemented for recovery.

The mismatch between fluid intakes and sweat losses in team sports is often more than one litre (two pints) and higher in hotter, humid conditions. That there is little evidence linking fluid imbalances with poor motor performance is only because it is difficult to measure. However, a study has shown that moderate levels of dehydration impair bowling accuracy in skilled cricket players.

Team and travel dynamics add to the nutrition demands of these sports. Foreign foods and food safety, monotony, food viewed as a treat, limited food choices, and individual preferences within the team are some of the common challenges that can be managed with a team approach.

NUTRITION GAME PLAN

You need an organized approach to nutrition at the beginning of each week, including a weekend plan if that is when you compete (*see Making a Plan pp44–57*). The specific energy systems (*see pp28, 148*) used in your sport and your training details (type, duration and frequency) need to be considered. Recovery after weekend competition is important, otherwise your training will be compromised in the following week.

HIGH ENERGY AND CARBOHYDRATE REQUIREMENTS

Carbo-loading (consuming up to 8–10g carbohydrate per kilogram body weight with an exercise taper) is not needed for a single training session or match (if shorter than 90 minutes). The amount of carbohydrate required will be determined by the amount and intensity of training (*see p46*). In tournaments, where multiple games may be played over a short period, this may need to be increased.

FLUID

You should have your own fluid-intake plan. You can use pre- and post-exercise body mass to estimate your fluid requirements and aim to keep the difference to less than 1kg (2.2 lb). Practise good drinking strategies in training by organizing access to your own drink bottle, ensuring that cool, palatable drinks are always available.

The rules of your sport, the environment (factors such as whether it is played in- or outdoors, uniforms, headgear) will determine your strategies. You should identify opportunities within the regulations and practices of your sport for frequent fluid intake (ideally every 10–15 minutes). (*For pre-, during and post-training fluid requirements, see p64.*)

Sports drinks containing carbohydrate provide both fluid and energy. In hotter environments and indoor sports like badminton, the addition of electrolytes can be beneficial. In tournament situations there may be inadequate time for complete recovery of fluid and fuel between games and the intake of a carbohydrate-rich sports drink during and after the game is essential. Caffeine-containing beverages and alcohol should not be taken immediately after exercise. When injured, the delay should be even longer. Alcohol is part of the culture of some sports and so creative strategies to reduce alcohol intake may be required (and better accepted). A beer shandy with low-alcohol beer is a better alternative to beverages with a higher alcohol content and less carbohydrate. (*See pp68–69 for other alcohol tips.*)

PROTEIN REQUIREMENTS

Many athletes resort to using protein supplements, creatine and HMB (*see p98*) to increase their muscle mass. Overuse of some supplements can be counterproductive and result in too much bulk and, ultimately, fat mass gain. These supplements should never be taken to replace dietary strategies.

Increased protein intakes, creatine and HMB supplementation may be of benefit to some athletes in these sports, but responses are individual. Athletes wanting to reduce body fat may be tempted to use fat-cutters, but they are ineffective and often unsafe (*see p100*).

RECOVERY

Implement strategies to promote speedy recovery from training and competition. Management and fitness trainers may need to ensure that appropriate recovery snacks and drinks are available in locker rooms and that the foods served at the grounds and functions meet the nutritional needs of the players. (*See Recovery Snacks p55*).

COMPETITION NUTRITION, TEAM
AND TRAVEL DYNAMICS

Competition nutrition should take into account the duration and intensity of the competition, the time-table, environmental conditions and travel. Timing of the pre-competition meal may be difficult in certain sports such as tennis and cricket, so you need to be adaptable, plan ahead and be prepared.

Eating together as a team will raise morale before a game and help focus for the game.

Menus should offer choices, acknowledge traditions and meet the nutrition requirements of individual team members, which may be very different to those of non-playing team members (management, for instance) and non-athletic guests. 'Menu fatigue' can be avoided with theme nights, restaurant meals (pre-organized menus) and barbecues to break the monotony. Since some athletes live in hotels and others in self-catering facilities on a budget, it must be determined in advance what cooking facilities and equipment are available. Recipes, basic ingredients and equipment (such as blenders) may need to be packed when travelling. (*For other ways to maximize nutrition while travelling, see pp56–57.*)

Sponsorship for any foods, drinks or supplements must be thoroughly assessed to ensure that these products are of benefit, safe and do not contain banned substances.

CASE STUDY
A CASE OF CHEAP ADVERTISING

BACKGROUND

Bokkie Strong,* an international rugby player aged 29 years, was married with two children and worked as an accountant. His weight was 101.2kg (223 lb); height 201cm (6ft, 7 in); sum of skinfolds 53.2mm; muscle mass 58.2kg (128 lb) and body fat 11.7%. He had no medical history and needed to gain 5kg (11 lb) of mainly muscle for his position of play – lock.

* Name changed to protect client confidentiality.

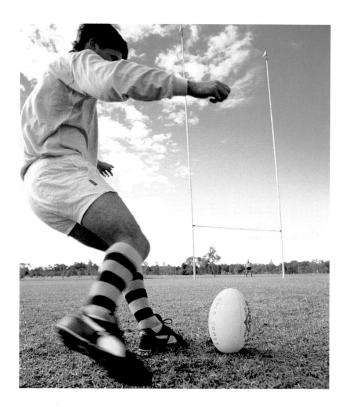

Above *Pre-competition dietary strategies sustain energy levels and concentration for the duration of the match.*
Opposite *Ensure that main meals always include lean protein.*

DIETARY AND TRAINING HISTORY

Mr Strong's current training was focused on aerobic fitness with very little resistance training. He had difficulty in gaining weight and lacked appetite, especially after training. A member of the management team was aware of his need to gain weight and offered him supplements from a network marketing company (at reduced rates) in return for using his 'newly constructed body' for advertising.

TYPICAL DAILY DIET

06:00	Banana or apple
08:00	250ml (1 cup) protein shake
10:00	4 breakfast wheat biscuits with milk
	3-egg omelette with ham, cheese and tomato
	2 slices toast with apricot jam
	250ml (8 fl oz) juice
12:00	250g (½ lb) meat with rice, sweet potato and carrots
19:00	2 packets of flavoured quick-cooking noodles
	500ml (2 cups) ice cream and fruit

RECOMMENDATIONS

MAIN CONCERNS

Mr Strong was not eating sufficient carbohydrate and protein to cover his training requirements and to allow for muscle growth. Infrequent meals with long gaps and missing out on recovery snacks and drinks also created a problem. Supper was disorganized, often lacking protein. Other concerns included business lunches, when he tended to make high-fat choices at the expense of carbohydrate and protein. His past approach to supplementation was haphazard and he was a soft target for cheap advertising with probably very little personal gain and the potential risk of unsafe supplements. His training regime also needed to be revised.

DIETARY ADVICE

To increase muscle mass, he needed to increase his intake of carbohydrate and protein-rich foods, and to add a recovery snack after training sessions. He also needed to ensure he had smaller, more frequent meals and snacks throughout the day, including a late-night snack. Carbohydrate intake could be increased with more fruit, juice, dried fruit as well as sandwiches, sports bars and fruit yoghurt.

A FEW QUICK AND EASY TIPS TO BOOST HIS PROTEIN INTAKE AT SUPPERTIME:

- crumbed chicken or fish (baked) with oven-baked chips and peas
- grilled chicken kebabs or chicken sausage served with rice or potato and vegetables (frozen or fresh)
- toast and scrambled eggs, tuna, baked beans and salad
- quick-cooking noodles, tuna, tomato, onion and salad
- pasta, low-fat lean mince in tomato sauce and a salad.

SUPPLEMENTS

The recommended dietary changes were already a step toward achieving his goal. He could top this up with a protein and carbohydrate supplement and creatine, according to the recommendations in chapter 7. He was advised to get the supplement manufacturing company to give him a certificate guaranteeing product purity, stating that they would accept liability if he tested positive for a banned substance. However, he was made aware that a once-off certificate did not guarantee purity of future batches of the product.

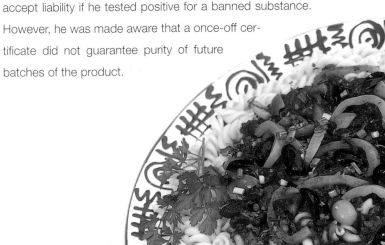

CASE STUDY

TEAM TACTICS

Parents needed to organize an eight-day cricket tour for the school's under-19 A-side. The plan was that the budget hotel would offer the full buffet for breakfast. Mothers would be responsible for providing lunches at the cricket grounds. For supper they would go to restaurants or fast-food outlets. They had been offered the sponsorship of a newly launched sports drink.

Additional Tips

Extra bread, fruit, juice, colddrinks and sports drinks to be provided.

Mothers had forgotten about tea breaks and the following items could be provided at the grounds: fruit, individual low-fat yoghurts, sports or breakfast bars, muffins and raisin buns, sandwiches with low-fat cheese, peanut butter and jam or honey.

BREAKFAST

Players were advised to select a variety of different carbohydrates and protein-rich (lower fat) items off the standard breakfast buffet menu to meet their individual requirements and preferences. This included cereals served with low-fat milk or yoghurt; a selection of bread and rolls with lean cold meats, low-fat cheese, peanut butter, jam and honey; fresh fruit and fruit juice. Hot items included porridge, eggs (boiled, poached or scrambled), baked beans, grilled tomatoes, mushrooms and flapjacks.

It was recommended that a low-fat meal replacement also be made available for players who were in the habit of skipping breakfast before batting or bowling 'to play light.'

LUNCH

The lunch menus drawn up by the catering committee are given in column A. Recommended changes are given in column B.

SUPPER

GENERAL GUIDELINES

They were advised to make reservations at the most suitable restaurants and to request menus in advance. Items could then be pre-selected to streamline orders. Extra rolls and bread could be ordered and a request made that sufficient water and colddrinks be available on all tables, since the conditions on tour were hot and humid.

Theme nights (Mexican, Chinese, Italian and a barbecue) could be organized for variety, (see pp50–51 for more ideas). When planning dinners, the lunch menu should be kept in mind to avoid repetition.

The performance-enhancing claims of the sponsored sports drink were impressive. Unfortunately, closer analysis showed that it contained large amounts of colourants, vitamins and minerals, but no carbohydrate. They were advised to seek sponsorship for a sports drink that contained carbohydrate and electrolytes.

A MENU AS DRAWN UP BY CATERING COMPANY	*B* RECOMMENDED CHANGES
DAY 1	
Chicken à la king and rice	Prepare with low-fat ingredients Add mixed peas and carrots
Coleslaw salad	Low-fat mayonnaise
Bread-and-butter pudding	Low-fat bread pudding with raisins and low-fat custard
DAY 2	
Tuna lasagne	Low-fat ingredients
Mixed salad	Dressing to be served separately
Apple pie with cream	Frozen yoghurt and fruit sorbets
DAY 3	
Grilled linefish with mixed vegetables	Fine
Parsley potatoes with garlic butter sauce	Oven-baked potato or sweet potato wedges
Crème caramel	Fruit-filled pancakes with ice cream
DAY 4	
Hungarian beef goulash served with butter noodles	Beef stir-fry with Chinese noodles
Mixed vegetables	Stir-fry vegetables
Mango mousse	Fine
DAY 5	
Cold cuts, breads, salads	Lean ham, shaved chicken and turkey, breads, salads
Fresh fruit salad	Fine
Swiss roll	Fine
DAY 6	
Open sandwiches and rolls with a variety of fillings	Tuna, egg, chicken (low-fat mayonnaise) and avocado
Trifle with cream	Jelly and custard

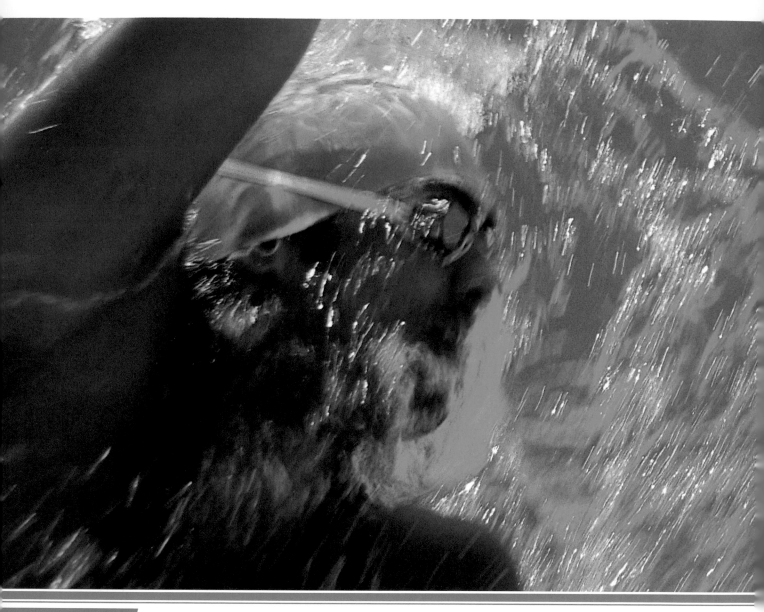

chapter 11

POWER, SPEED AND STRENGTH

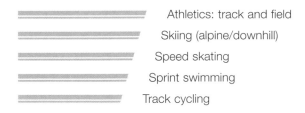

	Athletics: track and field
	Skiing (alpine/downhill)
	Speed skating
	Sprint swimming
	Track cycling

'He hadn't eaten all day ... all he was thinking about was a big plate of food to replace the energy he'd burnt up.' – Richard Williams about Linford Christie in *The View from the High Board*.

The sports in this category are all short in duration (from a 100m sprint run lasting less than 10 seconds to a 1500m swim lasting 15 minutes) and are performed at near maximal intensity. Competitors often participate in several short-duration events. Sprint distances and times vary according to the type of sport – a sprint swim in the Olympics is 50m, lasting about 21.8 seconds, speed skating is over 500m, lasting 36–40 seconds. A 50m sprint run takes less than 6 seconds, and the 100m less than 10 seconds. A track cyclist sprints 200m in about 10 seconds.

Success in these sports depends on the ability to generate power relative to body weight and to sustain peak power. While the maximum power output of any athlete depends on a number of factors, including body size, bigger is not always better. Power is the rate at which a given amount of exercise or work can be done. It is the force applied by an athlete, multiplied by the velocity of the movement, divided by the time taken to complete it. This power is largely generated anaerobically, requiring a maximal rate of energy expenditure that must be matched by a rapid rate of energy resynthesis (refuelling). For events lasting a few seconds, muscle ATP and creatine phosphate (CP) systems are the most important energy sources. In events lasting one minute, the contributions of energy from aerobic and anaerobic

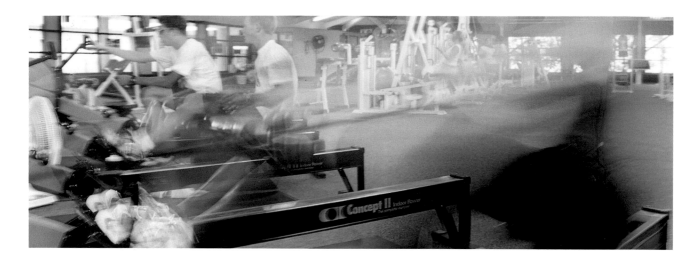

metabolism are equal. During these events, muscle fuel (glygogen) stores may not be depleted, and the major cause of fatigue is the build-up of hydrogen ions (H+), a by-product of anaerobic metabolism. In longer events aerobic metabolism becomes more important, but below 15 minutes it is unlikely that muscle glycogen stores will be depleted.

TRAINING FOR SPEED

For these events the quality of the training is far more important than the quantity. The core components of training need to include:

- a moderate base of aerobic conditioning and non-specific general fitness during the athletes' off-season
- attention to technique and specific drills during the pre-season training period
- extensive, year-round resistance and circuit training
- use of plyometrics and other forms of high-velocity resistance training to improve muscle power
- stretching and mobility exercises performed before and after most hard training sessions
- periodization of the training and racing programme.

Above *Aerobic conditioning needs to be maintained during the off-season.*

Opposite *Sprinters need power for a short time.*

Energy systems

The body uses four different energy systems to supply energy for different types of events. These energy systems do not switch on and off, but they always work together with one system predominating according to the intensity of effort (*see p28*).

EVENT DURATION	MAJOR ENERGY SYSTEMS USED	PRINCIPAL FUELS
6 seconds or less	Phosphagen	ATP and CP
30 seconds or less	Phosphagen, anaerobic glycolytic	ATP and CP, muscle glycogen
15 minutes or less	Anaerobic glycolytic, aerobic glycolytic	Muscle glycogen, blood glucose
15–60 minutes	Aerobic glycolytic	Muscle glycogen, blood glucose
60–90 minutes	Aerobic glycolytic, aerobic lipolytic	Muscle glycogen, blood glucose, intra-muscular fat
Longer than 90 minutes	Aerobic glycolytic, aerobic lipolytic	Muscle glycogen, blood glucose, intra- and extra-muscular fat

PHYSICAL DEMANDS AND CHARACTERISTICS

LOW BODY FAT LEVELS

Sprinters and jumpers typically share the low body fat levels of distance runners, since the power-to-weight ratio is an important determinant of performance. The most striking feature of elite sprinters is their muscular development, which allows them to generate high absolute power outputs for short periods of time.

In swimmers the relationship between body fat and body drag (resistance through the water, influenced by body size, the speed of swimming and other mechanical factors) is important. Above a critical percentage body fat, which may differ between individuals, an increase in body fat will increase body drag. Although increased body fat is likely to enhance buoyancy, the increase in body drag will offset any advantage resulting from improved buoyancy. Gender and event distance are two other factors which influence this relationship. Females have more fat than males, and distance swimmers generally have more body fat than sprint swimmers.

In cyclists the high ratio of muscle to fat enables them to maximize their force output. Any non-functional weight has various effects on cycling performance, which includes slowing the rate of acceleration, increasing the rolling resistance of the tyres, and increasing the frontal surface area.

MUSCLE FIBRE TYPE

Studies from the 1970s suggest that the best sprinters have a higher than average proportion of fast-twitch fibres (*see glossary*) in their leg muscles. Swimmers, however, are noted for their upper-body muscle development. Just as important as the quality of the muscle is the number of fast-twitch fibres that can be recruited during maximal exercise. The successful sprinter is able to use a greater proportion of their fast-twitch fibres compared to less well-trained athletes.

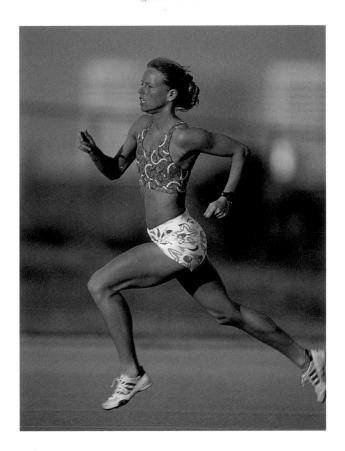

GENERAL

Athletes like elite sprinters, who compete in high-intensity events lasting less than 30 seconds, require the following characteristics to be successful:

- a high degree of muscularity
- limbs involved in propulsion are long (for leverage)
- a high proportion of fast-twitch fibres in the muscles involved in the activity
- the ability to recruit a large proportion of these fibres
- a fast reaction time
- the ability to generate and sustain high power outputs or speeds of movement
- a moderate aerobic power
- technique and biomechanics – for a track cyclist, for example, position on the bike is important; for a swimmer, technique or stroke mechanics play a role.

COMMON NUTRITION ISSUES
TRAINING, COMPETITION AND PERIODIZATION

The principle of training should be to adapt and train the various energy systems (*see pp28, 148*) appropriate to the event. Training for sprint events should avoid hours of endurance-type training, which would simply introduce residual fatigue. However, fuel will always be more taxed in training, and eating strategies must take this into account. Nevertheless you should never do anything new in an event that has not been tried out in training. In most of these sports, training varies with the phase of the season and includes an initial aerobic endurance base, followed by various anaerobic training sessions where single or multi-effort intervals are performed at different percentages of maximal work output. Peaking for competition involves a period of tapering; reducing the training load. Athletes may concentrate on peaking for 1–2 major competitions in the year.

CARBOHYDRATE

Matching carbohydrate intake to training remains a priority for sprint-type athletes, but requirements do not reach the levels of endurance athletes. Eating too little carbohydrate will deplete muscle and liver glycogen stores, thereby preventing optimal recovery and affecting training capacity on following days (*see p46*).

FLUID

Fluid intake during training is often neglected and all athletes should be encouraged to take their own sports drinks to training. It should be accessible, even in a sport like swimming when it is not always possible to climb out of the pool.

SUPPLEMENTS

Many supplements are sold on the premise of enhancing energy production via four commonly designated energy systems: the ATP-CP, lactic acid, aerobic glycolytic and aerobic lipolytic energy systems (*see pp28, 148*), for athletes

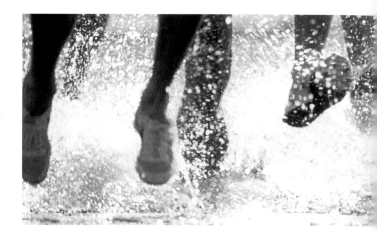

participating in sprint-type events. There is evidence that creatine and bicarbonate loading is useful, although individuals respond differently. However, there is currently little or no evidence to support the use of other supplements for which these claims are made.

NUTRITION GAME PLAN
COMPETITION NUTRITION

BEFORE — IS CARBO-LOADING REQUIRED?

Competition, often spread out over several days, usually comprises a number of short-duration events. There may be heats, semi-finals, finals and a qualifying round.

Since these events do not deplete muscle glycogen stores, there is no advantage in strict carbo-loading before a competition. The additional glycogen and water is simply extra weight to carry, and can therefore even be a disadvantage – especially in jumps and hurdles where you must lift yourself off the ground and propel yourself forward.

DURING —

COMPETITION-DAY FOOD AND FLUID INTAKE

The day of competition is best tackled with glycogen stores topped up to their usual resting level. With a high-carbohydrate diet already in place for training needs, glycogen levels can be restored before competition with 24–36 hours of rest or very light training. (*See chapter 3 for the role of the pre-competition meal.*)

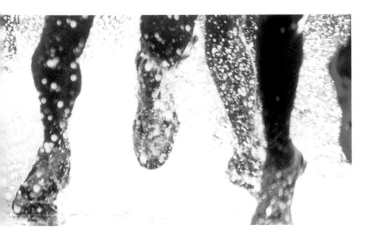

Choose a high-carbohydrate meal that suits the time of your event and your personal preference. If you are competing in a heat early in the morning, you may only have time for a light breakfast. Late afternoon and evening events may allow you to eat your usual breakfast, and even lunch, finishing off with a snack 2–3 hours before the event. Experiment in training if an important competition is coming up and you are scheduled to compete at an unaccustomed time. Drink plenty of fluids when you are competing in hot weather.

Your nutritional goals are to keep well hydrated and to maintain blood glucose levels. Plan your meals and snacks according to the time interval between events. Avoid getting hungry (and competing on an uncomfortably full stomach) by eating smaller, easily digestible foods that empty from the stomach quickly.

AFTER — RECOVERY

In a multi-event competition, your recovery plan will affect each subsequent event. To avoid gut discomfort, you will have to choose between solid foods or drinks, depending on the interval between events. Situations like a warm-down or celebrations may affect your recovery plan. You may also lack appetite or interest in food and choices at the venue may not be suitable to meet your needs. Plan ahead to have your recovery snacks and drinks accessible. (*For practical ideas and tips refer to the case study that follows and the general guidelines for recovery in chapter 3.*)

CASE STUDY

WATERLOGGED

BACKGROUND

Jay Seconds* was a 19-year-old national 100m and 200m sprinter. With a height of 1.86m (6ft 1 in), weight 84kg (185 lb), and sum of 7 skinfolds 34mm, he had 7.5% body fat. He had been taking creatine, but stopped because his weight increased, he was getting cramps, stiff joints, he felt inflexible and waterlogged. He had just started taking spirulina, and asked about the use of sodium phosphate, bicarbonate, ATP, a lactic acid buffer and a ribose supplement recommended by his coach to increase his speed and power.

* Name changed to protect client confidentiality.

DIETARY AND TRAINING HISTORY

Haphazard eating patterns was a key problem. Jay was skipping meals and often resorted to high-fat snacks at the track and gym, obviously missing out on much-needed carbohydrate and protein. He also did not pay much attention to his fluid intake. Jay trained six days a week, with a rest day on Sunday. In season, he increased gym training.

RECOMMENDATIONS

MAIN CONCERNS

Jay's coach was overly keen on supplements to improve performance, when many aspects of Jay's diet could easily be improved to the same effect. Some of the symptoms that he reported could be linked to creatine usage.

DIETARY ADVICE

The pros and cons of every supplement were discussed, so that Jay could make an informed decision based on scientific evidence (*see overleaf*).

Above left *Glycogen levels can be restored before competition with 24–36 hours of rest or very light training.*

SUPPLEMENTS FOR ENERGY
THE ATP-CP ENERGY SYSTEM

ATP is the immediate energy source for muscle contraction, while creatine phosphate (CP) provides for the rapid resynthesis of ATP (*see p97*). The ATP-CP energy system would be important for events involving explosive power during the final thrust.

During events such as shotput, discus, javelin, long jump, high jump and pole vault, 100 and 200m dashes, the 110m hurdles, and even longer events such as 400m races, it is important to achieve and maintain peak muscular force production. Since this may depend on the athlete's natural levels of ATP and CP, several nutrients have been used in an attempt to increase these levels or to enhance performance of the ATP-CP energy system in other ways.

THE NUCLEOTIDE ATP

ATP is composed of a base (adenosine), a sugar (ribose), and three high-energy phosphate bonds which are broken down during metabolism. It is contained in all body cells, where it plays a fundamental role in energy storage, transformation and release. It is given by mouth or by injection, but there is no evidence that it does what it purports to do, namely increase ATP levels in muscle.

CREATINE

There is strong evidence to support the use of creatine in sprint-type events (*see p97*). Some athletes do not derive benefit from using creatine ('non-responders') and the use of creatine is not a substitute for training and diet. There are also guidelines on how to best take creatine to avoid unwanted side effects (*see pp97–99*).

SUPPLEMENTS THAT DELAY
LACTIC ACID ACCUMULATION

As a result of anaerobic glycolysis, lactic acid accumulates and is popularly associated with the onset of fatigue and the 'burning' feeling that accompanies fatigue and exhaustion during or just after maximal exercise. However, this is not the case and it is the production of hydrogen ions (H^+) (and thus the rise in muscle acidity), which interferes with muscle contractility and inhibits further high-intensity exercise. The goal is thus to buffer these H^+ ions. The use of sodium bicarbonate or sodium citrate supplements may be useful, rather than a supplement that will delay the accumulation of lactic acid. Sodium bicarbonate and citrate can only be taken in the form of a supplement, since it is not available as food (*see p103*).

RIBOSE

This is a pentose carbohydrate used in the manufacture of ATP. It is sold in tablet form, which is well absorbed from the gut. The theory behind its use is that it can enhance performance by increasing the rate of ATP regeneration. However, there is no evidence that it is incorporated by the body into ATP and, although manufacturers claim many trials have been performed, no evidence exists that it has any effect on athletic performance.

SPIRULINA

There is no published scientific evidence that spirulina improves athletic performance and the estimated effect on performance is zero.

ADVICE ON SUPPLEMENTS

Jay was encouraged to correct his diet before considering supplements, especially since he could now see that these supplements were not addressing his real problem i.e. lack of carbohydrate and protein. Once his diet was improved, he could then reconsider using creatine, provided this was taken according to current guidelines and that he understood that, as with all supplements, safety and purity issues remained a concern.

CASE STUDY
DAY AT THE TRACK

BACKGROUND

Sue Long* was a 17-year-old track athlete. She participated in the long jump and pole vaulting events. Her current weight was 52.7kg (116 lb), muscle mass 25.7kg (56.7 lb), body fat 20.5% and sum of 7 skinfolds 74.7mm. She battled on race days with vomiting, low blood glucose levels and fatigue, and wanted to know whether carbo-loading would improve her performance.

* Name changed to protect client confidentiality.

DIETARY AND TRAINING HISTORY

She was training about 10 hours a week, which included running, strength training and technique. Dietary assessment showed a low energy intake, with insufficient carbohydrate and protein to cover training demands. Her dietary fat intake was low and she drank plenty of water.

The night before competition she ate pasta with a fresh tomato topping and generally ate nothing during the competition, but drank about 500ml (1pt) water per hour. If hungry after competing, she would eat what she liked and this typically included burgers, pies and hot chips, or whatever was available at the stadium.

RECOMMENDATIONS

MAIN CONCERNS AND DIETARY ADVICE

Sue Long's fluid intake lacked carbohydrate and electrolytes, which are not only important when competing in high temperatures, but also an important component of fluid intake when lacking appetite or feeling anxious about eating.

For the type of event in which she was competing, carbohydrate loading was not necessary and could increase body weight. Once her training diet had been optimized, all she needed to do before the competition was to sustain her diet and rest, or train lightly for the next 24–36 hours. For multiple events spread over a day, she was encouraged to rehydrate and refuel between events.

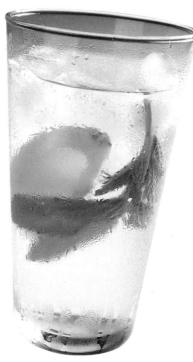

Low-fat liquid meal replacements kept cool on ice in a cooler bag would be useful if she lacked appetite before competition. This would be better than the high-fat foods available at the stadium. She also needed to take recovery snacks to the competition (*see p55*).

Special strategies for competing in hot environments were discussed. She was advised to include sports drinks and salty snacks (pretzels and salty crackers) and to keep cool by staying in the shade.

Fatigue could only be dealt with once it was established whether she experienced it only on competition days, and factors such as inadequate carbohydrate and iron intakes had been excluded (*see Sports Anaemia p78*).

Her day-to-day training diet needed to provide more energy, carbohydrate and protein, but had to be introduced gradually as she feared weight gain. To prevent this she could concentrate on low-fat high-fibre food on training days and limit her intake of concentrated calories as found in sports drinks and cold drinks. She could try sports waters, since these contain virtually no calories but still provide electrolytes. Sue was encouraged to keep a food diary as this would help identify areas in the diet that could still be improved and would also help her keep on track.

Above *Special strategies are required when competing in a hot environment.*

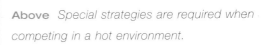

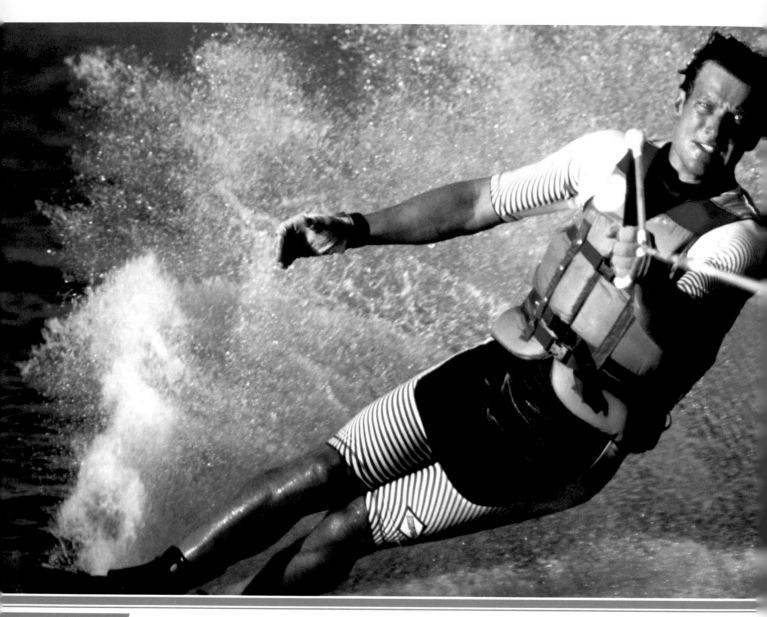

chapter 12

SKILL, CONCENTRATION AND MANOEUVRES

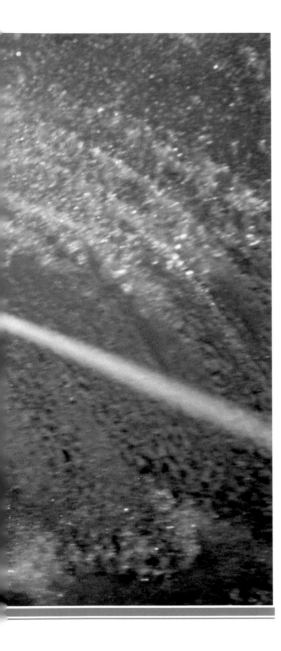

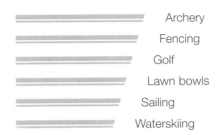
Archery
Fencing
Golf
Lawn bowls
Sailing
Waterskiing

All these sports require tactical and technical skills as well as balance and agility. Environmental conditions, equipment and clothing vary in these sports.

'I'm about a buck80 (180 lb) and my percentage of body fat is a bogey on a par 4, so while there is still room for improvement I've done a decent job of putting on the right kind of weight. But more importantly, my energy level and stamina are the highest since I was a kid. I attribute it to watching what and when I eat.' – Tiger Woods *How I Play Golf,* 2001

PHYSICAL DEMANDS AND CHARACTERISTICS

Training for most of these sports involves many hours, often outdoors in adverse environmental conditions. The environment affects nutritional demands – sailing in hot and windy conditions will often deplete a sailor's reserves of fuel. Clothing, indoors or outdoors, affects fluid requirements. Fencers wear a jacket, pants, plaston (underarm protection), socks, a mask and glove, so that only the trailing hand and the back of the head are exposed, limiting heat dissipation. Archers wear tight-fitting clothing and compete in several rounds in varying temperatures.

Training for those sports focuses on strength and aerobic endurance, flexibility to minimize the risk of injury, skills to handle equipment, and tactics (wind tactics and boat-to-boat tactics in sailing, for instance). Each class of sailing requires a different set of skills and makes different physical demands, which also vary depending on the position of the sailor in the boat.

Success in these sports often relies on the ability to concentrate fully, sometimes over many days. The current Olympic format for sailing involves 12 races sailed over 11 days, with one lay day (no racing). Two races are scheduled each day and the sailor is expected to stay out on the water between races. Races vary in length from 45 to 105 minutes.

Blood sugar levels and dehydration affect skill and concentration, so nutritional strategies must optimize these. Although there are many height and weight ranges for these sports, in most cases a low sum of skinfolds (see p126) is desirable. This decreases the susceptibility to fatigue, which can lead to loss of skill and concentration. In sailing, the ideal anthropometric and physical characteristics depend on the class and event – some sailors may deliberately try to gain or lose weight.

COMMON NUTRITION ISSUES
ENVIRONMENT

Energy and fluid requirements will depend on whether the sport is practised indoors or outdoors. Indoors, fluid requirements are increased, and more so when wearing protective clothing (as in fencing). Competing outdoors in extreme temperatures will also increase fluid requirements. Sailing in strong wind will increase energy requirements, while rough weather and sea conditions may affect appetite.

COMPETITION AND TRAINING

All competition strategies should be tried and tested in training. The stress of competition may result in a lack of appetite, diarrhoea and weight loss. Diarrhoea in turn affects fluid and electrolyte balance, which should be treated with rehydration formulae. Stress increases the requirements for the water-soluble vitamins B and C at a time when fruit and vegetable intake may also be poor. Stress relief through alcohol consumption and cigarette smoking also increase your requirements for these vitamins.

VISION

The environment affects eye health and the eyes also need to be nourished. The sun's glare on water, air pollution and cigarette smoke in clubhouses can cause eye irritation and fatigue. Alcohol affects focus, causes blurred vision, and reduces peripheral vision. Heavy drinking impedes the muscular reflexes controlling most visual skills. A deficiency of vitamin A is strongly associated with night blindness and reduced ability to adjust from darkness to light and back.

The sun's glare on water and lights in sport arenas causes the eye to rapidly burn up large amounts of vitamin A, which will need to be replenished (see Food Sources p158).

Healthy, nourished eyes react faster to visual stimuli, so a good diet is essential for building good eye skills, preventing

FOOD ITEM
Espresso
Brewed/percolated coffee, drip coffee
Instant coffee
Tea
Green tea
Hot chocolate
Maté (South American herb, chewed or taken as a drink)
Chocolate bar (milk)
Chocolate bar (dark)
Chocolate brownie
Carbonated beverages (including many diet drinks)
Red Bull Energy Drink
Iced Tea – some brands
Powerbar caffeinated power gel
Gu caffeinated sports gel

and even curing a number of visual problems. There are several nutrition strategies linked with better eyesight, higher levels of acuity, reduced fatigue and the improvement of many ocular functions (*see p158*).

CONCENTRATION

Psychological factors such as arousal and anxiety levels, which affect performance, can be modified by nutritional practices. For example, supplements of vitamin B_1, B_6 and B_{12} (rapidly depleted during periods of tension and stress) have been found to improve firing accuracy in pistol shooting. However, before specific practical advice can be given, more research is needed on other supplements such as choline, amino acids, ginseng, other herbals and adaptogens (for

example, eleutherococcus) and some of the antioxidants that are said to alleviate fatigue and improve stamina.

Caffeine also increases arousal, but as a central nervous system stimulant it can be counterproductive by also increasing nervousness, anxiety, and causing palpitations, headaches and dehydration (*see p100*). Find out which foods and drinks contain caffeine – these include energy and sports drinks, tea, coffee, sports gels and drugs (caffeine is an ingredient in more than 1000 over-the-counter drugs and prescription drugs) to avoid undesirable side effects.

OTHER NOT-SO-OBVIOUS SOURCES OF CAFFEINE INCLUDE:

many non-prescription medications (pain killers, cold, headache and weight-loss preparations)

herbs and tonics (Guarana, Paullinia cupana)

fat-cutting/weight loss/energy supplements

herbals (e.g. Biolean) and tonics

bottled waters (e.g. Buzz Water)

chewing gum (e.g. Stay-A-Lert)

kola nut (cola acuminata).

TIPS ON REDUCING CAFFEINE INTAKE

- Cut back gradually to avoid headaches and other symptoms of sudden caffeine withdrawal.
- Mix decaffeinated and caffeinated coffee.
- Drink a latte with more low-fat milk than coffee.
- Brew tea for less time.
- Opt for other beverages, such as herbal teas or milk.
- Drink juice instead of cola.
- Avoid caffeine later in the day.
- Drink smaller quantities at a time.

SERVING	CAFFEINE [MG]
60ml (¼cup)	100
250ml (1 cup)	80–135 and more
250ml (1 cup)	60 (12–169)
250ml (1 cup)	27 (9–51)
250ml (1 cup)	35
250ml (1 cup)	5–10
200ml (⅔ cup)	25–150
60g (2 oz)	5–15
60g (2 oz)	10–50
1 average	8
340ml (11 fl oz)	40–55
250ml (1 cup)	80
340ml (11 fl oz)	70
40g (1⅛ oz) sachet	25
32g (1 oz)	20

Left *The caffeine content of various foods and drinks is not always obvious.*

NUTRITION GAME PLAN
BE PREPARED – PLAN AHEAD OF TIME

Be practical – if unsuitable food is on offer at venues, take food, snacks and drinks along in insulated containers. Sailors should ensure that the support craft carries enough food and drink. When travelling, ensure that accommodation bookings are conveniently located and close to shops and restaurants. This will also help your budget. Forward planning will prevent unnecessary stress and give you a psychological advantage.

You should establish eating patterns that promote long-term health, with variety, balance and moderation.

CHOOSE FOODS THAT SUSTAIN CONCENTRATION

Modifying the type of carbohydrate in the diet can help athletes involved in endurance sports, or who require immense concentration skills over time.

Carbohydrates have traditionally been ranked according to their nutrient density with the more complex carbohydrates (starches made up of thousands of sugar molecules joined together) achieving higher scores than the simple carbohydrates (sugars of one or two molecules).

Recent research has compared individual carbohydrate foods according to their overall effects on blood sugar levels, a system referred to as the Glycaemic Index (GI) (*see p 17*). Different foods (each providing 50g of carbohydrate) have been tested under the same conditions, using either pure glucose or white bread as a reference. With pure glucose as a reference (giving it a GI value of 100, since it causes a high blood glucose response), foods are ranked as follows: high GI foods (value over 70), moderate GI foods (55–70) and low GI foods (under 55). (*See GI table p85.*)

There are several factors that affect the GI of foods and these include the way in which complex carbohydrate molecules are joined, the physical form of the food (whether it is thick and sticky, in whole pieces or mashed up, hot or cold), and the presence of other components such as soluble fibre,

sugar, protein, fat, phytates and tannins. This is why foods often have a higher (or lower) GI than expected. The GI of wheat biscuits, for example, is pushed up because, after processing, the fibre is no longer intact.

SLOW OR FAST ENERGY FIX
PRACTICAL POINTERS

1. During the day, to sustain energy levels and keep hunger at bay, go for low GI foods.
2. Pre-exercise – go for low GI foods if you tend to suffer the blood glucose roller coaster after consuming pre-event carbohydrates. To avoid gastrointestinal discomfort, choose those lower in fibre and residue.
3. During and after exercise (especially if exercising for longer than 90 minutes) – go for moderate to high GI foods.

FOCUS ON EYE NUTRITION

1. Ensure adequate dietary intakes of vitamins B and C by consuming a wide variety of different foods that provide good sources of these vitamins (see pp24, 26).
2. Eat foods rich in vitamin A (liver, fish oils, milk and butter) if you are exposed to bright lights and glare. Beta carotene, the pro-vitamin that the body converts to vitamin A, is found in yellow and orange fruit and vegetables (apricots, mangoes, carrots, sweet potatoes and squashes).
3. Another antioxidant that may protect against free radical damage caused by light exposure is vitamin E. Include cold-pressed seed oils, and avocados in your diet.
4. Vitamin supplements need to be used with discretion. Vitamin A is a fat-soluble vitamin, which can become toxic if taken in excess. Do not exceed the Daily Upper Limit of 3000µg per day (above 19 years).
5. Limit alcohol consumption and if you do drink you may need to supplement your diet with extra amounts of vitamins B and C, the two most depleted by alcohol.

CASE STUDY

FAT CIRCUIT

BACKGROUND

Mr Chip Davis* was a 36-year-old golfer who played most of his tournaments on the summer circuit, but played in Europe during the winter months. While on tour he ate out at restaurants six nights a week and while travelling he snacked on high-fat foods. He was keen to lose weight and improve his golf performance, but was concerned that losing weight would change his swing.

His weight was 88.8kg (196 lb), height 1.90m (6ft 3in), sum of 7 skinfolds 142.2mm and body fat 23.9%. His current Total Cholesterol (TC) level was 7mmol/ℓ (280mg/dl). There was a strong family history of heart disease and his father had died at the age of 33.

* Name changed to protect client confidentiality.

DIETARY AND TRAINING HISTORY

BREAKFAST
Toasted muesli with full-cream milk

LUNCH
Toasted cheese and hot chips

Coke

OR a Roquefort OR Caesar salad with Coke

SUPPER
Pasta (Alfredo)

OR home-barbecued lamb chops with jacket potato

OR hot dogs, McDonalds or Mexican-style take-outs

SNACKS
Banana

Peanut butter bars

Bagel with cream cheese

Brownies

Alcohol – every second night before supper 2–3 glasses of wine

RECOMMENDATIONS

MAIN CONCERNS

There is no scientific evidence to show that overweight golfers will improve their game with weight loss, but there are other benefits such as improved heat tolerance, endurance and fitness. This helps to prevent fatigue which, in turn, will affect skill and concentration.

In this case there was some concern because fat around the abdomen increases the risk of cardiovascular disease.

DIETARY ADVICE

Small changes would go a long way to improve Chip's game and long-term health. These needed to be made gradually so that he could monitor his performance and make the necessary adjustments to his game.

Decreasing his intake of dietary fat and cholesterol could easily be achieved by making the following changes:

- Decreasing his total fat intake, especially from animal sources (full-cream milk, cheese, fatty meat and cream).
- At the half-way house, choosing untoasted sandwiches with lower fat fillings, chicken or tuna with low-fat mayonnaise, cottage cheese instead of cream cheese.
- Avoid doubling up on fat (skip margarine when using mayonnaise); use low-fat salad dressings or balsamic vinegar.
- Shifting to lower fat snacks such as fruit or cereal bars, which are portable and can be packed into the golf bag. Also ensure sufficient fluid intakes.
- Identifying restaurants that offer low-fat choices and avoid large portions of animal protein. Best Mexican choices include plenty rice with beans, with a tortilla or fajita (no cheese or sour cream) served with salsa and guacomole. (*For more ideas on restaurant meals – see guide pp50–51.*)

Although alcohol may improve HDL-cholesterol and be beneficial, it should not be used 'therapeutically' as the additional calories all add up and contribute to weight gain.

He was advised to have his cholesterol levels checked again in three months to review the need for intervention.

CASE STUDY
BARELY HOLDING ON

BACKGROUND

Mr John Matelot* was a professional Olympic Finn sailor who found it very challenging to gain weight, which would be advantageous for the physical exertion required to command his craft, especially for the hiking position (leaning out) in high wind speeds. His weight was 88kg (194 lb), height 1.85m (6ft 1in) with a sum of 7 skinfolds of 50mm. For several years, he had been following a lacto-ovo vegetarian diet (including milk and cheese, but excluding all other sources of animal protein). He had a history of anaemia, complained of always being tired and often sleeping the afternoon away. During competition, by the second day he would battle to keep going and also found that his concentration waned. He had limited cooking skills and when travelling relied heavily on take-outs, especially Chinese foods and pizza. When he successfully gained weight in the past, it was by taking creatine in combination with a gym programme and protein shakes. However, this lasted only one month, after which he got flu and then battled to regain the weight lost. The pressure was building up as the Olympics were not far away.

* Name changed to protect client confidentiality.

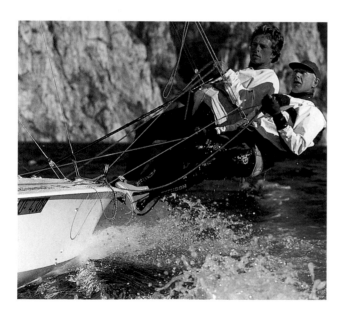

DIETARY AND TRAINING HISTORY

NON-RACE DAY

BREAKFAST 07:30

Coffee (no sugar)

2 bowls cereal with fat-free milk

1 fruit

LUNCH 13:00

Fruit

4–6 slices bread

Fillings would vary, but included cheese, egg, avocado pear, jam and peanut butter

SUPPER

Pasta, rice or potato and plenty of vegetables

DAILY EXTRAS

2 glasses vegetable or fruit juice

4–6 glasses water

1 sports drink

2 cartons of drinking yoghurt

Sometimes energy bars when training

He also ate nuts twice a week and chocolate once a week

RACE DAYS

On race days, breakfast would be the same. Prior to race departure he ate pasta, power bars, bread with salad fillings, bananas and supplements (spirulina and echinacea). He recently stopped taking creatine and the sporadic use of multivitamins. Previously, he has had iron and B_{12} injections.

TRAINING

He trained 3–4 hours on the water under different conditions every day, with at least an hour in the gym or running.

Left *Environmental conditions may affect appetite and increase energy and fluid requirements.*

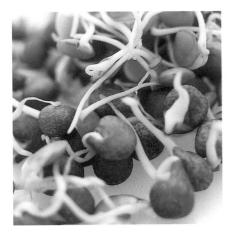
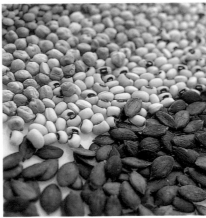
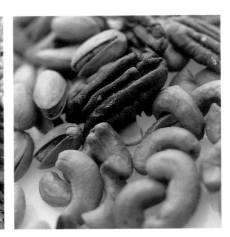

RECOMMENDATIONS

MAIN CONCERNS

There were many dietary factors that affected his recovery, therefore contributed to the build-up of fatigue in training and competition. A key concern was that his total energy intake was inadequate to cover his training needs and certainly not enough to allow for anabolic growth. Protein intake was too low and his protein choices were not good sources of iron. Because he was only eating three times a day, it was difficult to achieve his carbohydrate goals. He was not including additional carbohydrate via fluid.

His current supplement regime (although providing him with micronutrients) was not contributing calories and thus not helping him to increase his lean body mass.

DIETARY ADVICE

1. He needed to plan for six meals a day, of which three could be portable snacks.
2. Protein should be included at all meals:
   - At the main meal protein could be from beans, lentils, chickpeas, textured vegetable protein and tofu.
   - Extra milk or yoghurt drinks should be taken as snacks, fortified with skim milk powder.
   - Sandwich fillings should be protein-based: cheese with avocado and peanut butter combined with jam. He could explore other protein spreads and toppings like hummus, baked beans and felafel balls.
3. Snacks: nuts and raisins were encouraged as his percentage body fat was low. Mixed bars (protein and carbohydrate) and carbohydrate drinks would also help to boost his energy intake.
4. More fresh and dried fruit should be included, which would help to increase his vitamin intake.

If he focused on these dietary changes he could diminish his reliance on supplements, which was not getting to the core issues. Once these recommendations were implemented he could reconsider the use of creatine. Iron and vitamin B_{12} would need ongoing monitoring.

When competing he should add some protein to his carbohydrate-based meal, which would lower the GI and sustain energy levels. He was also encouraged to ensure an adequate stock of carbohydrate-rich bars and drinks.

Above left *Sprouts are low in calories and can be a good source of iron, and vitamins B and C.*
Above centre *Legumes are a good source of protein when combined with cereals/grains or nuts/seeds or dairy products.*
Above right *Nuts contain protein, but also fat.*

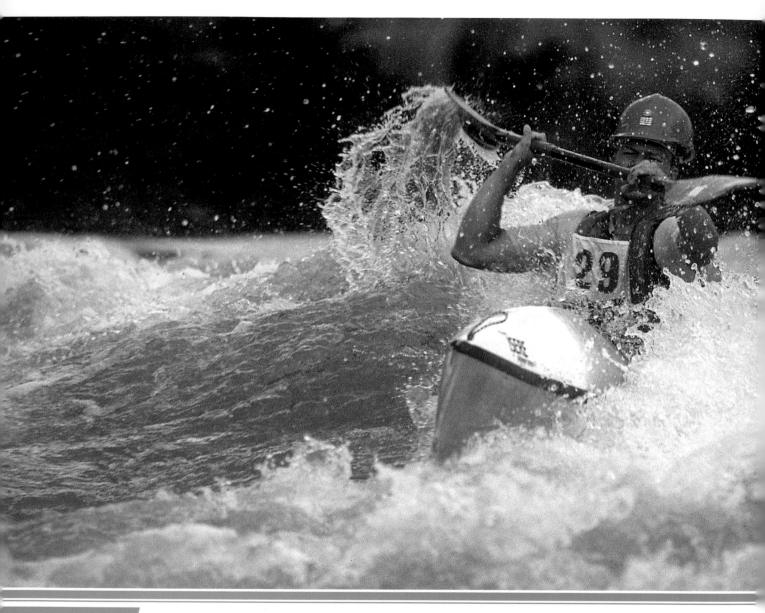

chapter 13

ADVENTURE AND EXTREME

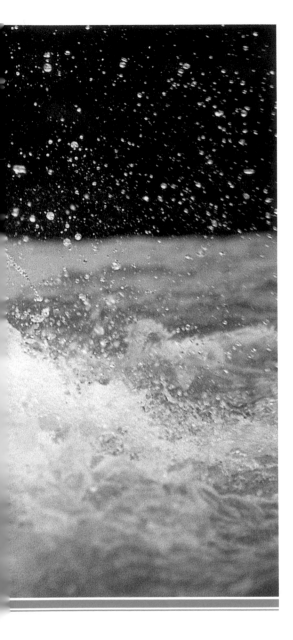

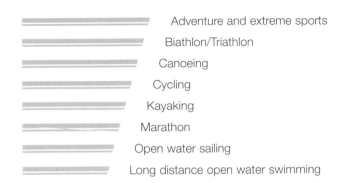

Adventure and extreme sports
Biathlon/Triathlon
Canoeing
Cycling
Kayaking
Marathon
Open water sailing
Long distance open water swimming

'*Now that I was finally here, ... I had no energy to care.*'
– John Krakauer, *Into Thin Air*, 1996.

The nutrition beliefs and practices of early marathoners and ultra-distance athletes were very different from those of today. Training and running 'tough' with little fuel and fluid was an acceptable practice even up until 1969, while open water sailors believed that the more emaciated you were, the more you had 'endured'.

In his book *Mind Over Matter*, Ranulph Fiennes describes his and Mike Stroud's diet in their epic 97-day manhaul crossing of the Antarctic continent in 1992/93. Even on 23,184kJ (5520kcal) per day each, a diet consisting of butter, cocoa, chocolate, cereal, soup, a freeze-dried meal and vegetables and a flapjack bar, each lost about 22kg (49 lb), more than half of that in muscle. Their dietary approach was more scientific than the unsuccessful, unassisted Antarctic crossings of others, but the battering that their bodies endured surely begs the question whether their diet was optimal.

With the advent of the muscle biopsy technique, more research on marathon runners became available, but for extreme sports and ultra-endurance events, research remained limited. Nutritional practices were often kept a secret as most of the evidence was anecdotal or the athletes were reluctant to reveal what they were doing because it was 'against traditional lore'.

These sports have become extremely popular, with an explosion in the types of events on offer. As a result there is a growing interest and need for more research specific to these sports. Products have been developed to include a wider range of better-tasting freeze-dried foods (from complete meals to desserts) as well as a range of compact, light and long-lasting nutrient-rich supermarket foods.

It is critical to match the nutrition requirements of a specific event to the physiological demands and practical limitations. In many of these events, stocking up at a local convenience store is not an option – you may be in the middle of an ocean or in a remote mountain range. Poor attention to nutrition on expeditions can thus be a costly affair – not only the financial cost of abandoning the expedition, but also in lives.

As the duration of an event increases, so does the role and benefits of nutrition. In all these sporting events your endogenous fuel reserves are stretched to the limit and your success depends on fuel reserves and fuel on hand. With careful dietary manipulation, fuel reserves can be maximized before the start and a good plan can keep these reserves topped up throughout the event.

The nutritional approach for these sports will vary according to the type of event and the level to which it is pursued. A standard marathon, ultra-marathon, road cycle race, an expedition where you carry your own food (manhauling) at high altitude, long-distance swimming, sailing and canoeing, hiking, mountaineering, rock climbing and kayaking all have different nutrition demands. Energy requirements for the ultra-endurance events can be as high as 33,600kJ (8000kcal). Food and meals become a highlight and need special attention to help alleviate unnecessary stress.

ENDURANCE

The standard marathon covers a distance of 42.2km (26.2 miles), with the top runners completing this distance in just over two hours. These runners, typically, are small and have low body fat levels, an advantage when body weight has to be carried over many kilometres and body temperature needs to be regulated, especially in hot and humid weather.

The nutritional advice given to marathon runners has gone from one extreme to the other. In the 1900s the advice was: 'Don't get into the habit of drinking and eating in a marathon race; some prominent runners do, but it is not beneficial.'

In 1996 the American College of Sports Medicine (ACSM) guidelines for fluid ingestion during exercise recommended: 'Runners should be encouraged to replace their sweat losses or consume 150–300ml (¼–⅔pt) every 15 minutes, which works out to 600–1200ml (1–2½pt) per hour.'

Following reports relating the deaths of marathon runners to water intoxication (hyponatraemia of exercise), the USA Track and Field have adopted new fluid guidelines of 400–800ml (¾–1½pt) per hour, but less for slower and smaller athletes exercising in mild environments. This differentiates between the size and speed of athletes and the environmental conditions (in colder temperatures, you need to drink less).

The one-size-fits-all approach resulted in, for example a female who runs 42km (26 miles) at less than 8–9km/hr (5–5½ miles/hr) – and consumes 300ml (⅔pt) every 15 minutes – drinking twice the required amount of fluid. This would have put her at risk of developing hyponatraemia. In longer events hyponatraemia becomes even more of a problem as there are more opportunities to drink.

Fluid is also a vehicle for much needed carbohydrate and electrolytes during these endurance events. A carbohydrate intake of 50–60g/hr is recommended. Try out different concentrations of sports drinks, gels with water and sports bars. Be cautious of concentrations greater than 10% because they may reduce gastric emptying, causing discomfort

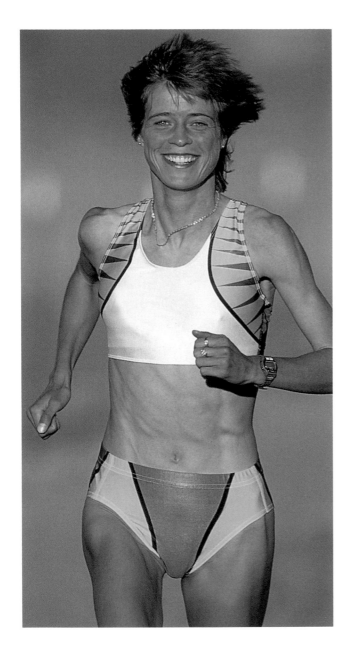

Above *Low body fat levels are an advantage for marathon runners, who need to carry their body weight over many kilometres.*
Right *Use clothing and equipment to store food and fluid.*

(*see p83*). 700ml (1½pt) of a typical sports drink at a concentration of 7% will provide 50g carbohydrate per hour and 20mmol/ℓ of sodium (*see p66 Osmolality*). This sodium concentration is less than sweat losses and so it is necessary to eat salty foods after the marathon as part of your recovery strategy.

CARBO-LOADING

For endurance events (all events lasting longer than 90 minutes) you need to maximize your muscle glycogen stores:

- Three days before the event (when your training should be tapered), consume 8–10g carbohydrate/kg body weight. For a 50kg (110 lb) athlete this means consuming 400–500g carbohydrate per day and for a 70kg (154 lb) athlete 560–700g carbohydrate per day
- Use the 50g carbohydrate list (*see p17*) to calculate quantities and to select preferred foods
- Carbohydrate must form the bulk of all meals and snacks
- Fluids and concentrated sources of carbohydrate can be used to ensure you meet your target
- Over the last 24 hours you can reduce the fibre and bulk of the diet to 'race light'
- 2–3 hours before the event have a light pre-event meal (*see p53*).

HOW DIFFERENT IS IT FOR CYCLISTS?

Pockets in cycling jerseys or bum bags for storing food, camel backs and bottle cages for carrying fluid make it easier for the cyclist to consume food and fluid 'on the run'. This allows greater variety as the cyclist can carry bananas, sports bars, dried fruit and sweets.

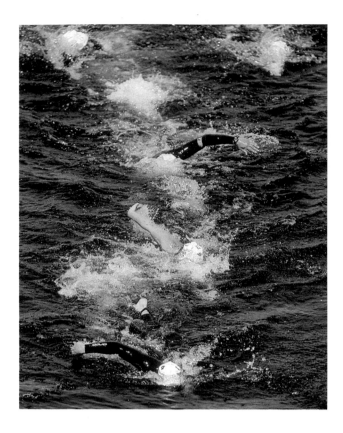

ULTRA-ENDURANCE

In ultra-endurance (events lasting longer than four hours, such as ultra-marathons, road cycle races and the Ironman triathlon), carbohydrate remains a limiting factor. Several strategies to increase fat oxidation have been tried, including the intravenous infusion of fat, the consumption of high-fat diets as well as the use of some drugs like heparin combined with a high fat intake. Following a study that showed performance benefits using medium chain triglycerides (MCT oils) in combination with carbohydrate, the use of MCTs became popular among some ultra-endurance athletes.

MCTs provide about 34kJ/g (8kcal/g) – almost like fat – and are more rapidly absorbed than longer chain fats, thus providing an additional and more efficient source of fuel. However, the performance benefits have not been replicated in other studies and the side effect of diarhhoea may adversely affect performance.

Tips for ultra-endurance events

1. If you decide to fat-load, your diet should increase to 60–70% fat for five days. This means including foods like chocolates, cream, full-cream milk, high-fat crackers and cheese.

2. Follow this with 1–3 days of carbo-loading (*see diet plan in case study p177*). Substitute all the high-fat foods with carbohydrate-rich foods (pasta, potatoes, bread, sugar, carbohydrate powders and bars) and carbohydrate drinks.

3. On the day of the event, start off with a light carbohydrate breakfast (porridge, low-fat yoghurt, pasta).

4. During the event ensure that you consume 40–60g of carbohydrate per hour. Popular choices are plain biscuits, bananas, pretzels, potatoes, salty soup, concentrated carbohydrate drinks and gels.

5. Don't be overzealous with fluid. Hyponatraemia (low blood sodium levels), which is potentially fatal, can result from water intoxication. Keep the stomach volume full by regularly topping up. Electrolytes such as sodium and potassium are lost in sweat. Depending on the environment you may need to consume 400–800mg sodium/hour in the form of electrolyte powders in a solution or real food (salty soup, pretzels, bananas for potassium). Electrolyte pills can also be used. These can be taken every hour to cover the losses of sodium chloride in sweat and urine, depending on the conditions. The hotter the ambient temperature, the more salt is needed.

6. Aid your recovery by consuming plenty of high GI carbohydrates afterward (sweets, pretzels, sports drinks, water biscuits, pancakes and syrup). You can add low-fat proteins.

(**For other strategies such as glycerol hyperhydration, see p67.*)

FREQUENTLY ASKED QUESTIONS AND ANSWERS ON FAT-LOADING

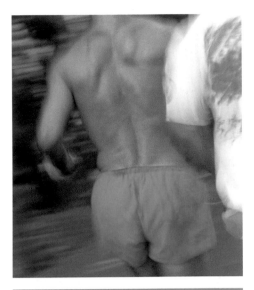

Which athletes can benefit from this regime?

Only well-trained athletes in ultra-endurance events (more than four hours) may benefit. Individual responses vary and these strategies should therefore be rehearsed during training and before a major competition. In some situations it can be impossible to complete the event on a high-carbohydrate diet because of the bulkiness, low-energy content and chewing time when compared to eating fat.

Are carbohydrates completely ruled out?

No, the high-fat diet of five days must be followed by 1–3 days of carbohydrate loading.

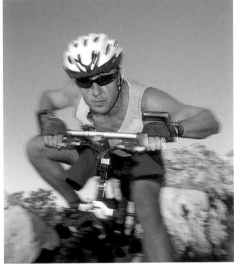

What type of fat should be consumed?

To get the desired effect of sparing the limited carbohydrate reserves, saturated (animal) fat, often referred to as 'bad' fats, should dominate the diet.

Will fat-loading cause weight gain or are there health risks associated with following a high-fat diet in the short term?

Studies to date have shown that this kind of diet does not alter weight, body fat or blood fat (cholesterol) levels.

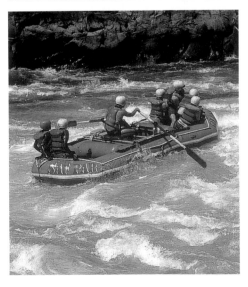

Opposite *Fluid remains a consideration, even during long-distance swims.*
Top, right *In hot environments, more salt is needed.*
Centre, right *High GI carbohydrates are a good source of fuel that can be taken during an event.*
Right *Eating for recovery should start as soon as possible after the event.*

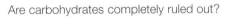

MULTISTAGE CYCLE EVENTS
(TOUR DE FRANCE, EPIC CYCLE TOUR)

Tour de France cyclists must pedal about 4000km (2486 miles) over a period of three weeks with only one day allowed for rest. The course includes 30 mountain passes, the highest of which reaches an altitude of about 2700m (8860ft). It is considered the most strenuous endurance competition.

In a study that examined the food intake and energy expenditure of five cyclists during this 22-day race, the energy expenditure per day was estimated to range from 25,400kJ (6060kcal) to 32,700kJ (7800kcal). The riders did well in balancing their energy needs on a daily basis over this period. This was important, since the large amounts required to be eaten would be hard to catch up from one day to the next if intake fell behind. There is only so much that you can put into your stomach each day.

The cyclists consumed 12–13g carbohydrate/kg body weight during the race – 30% from carbohydrate-rich fluid. Protein intake was more than adequate at over 3g/kg. Although they could have eaten more fat, only 23% of their energy was from fat, probably because of the possibility of gastric disturbances during high-intensity exercise. Nearly 60% of the total carbohydrate intake was consumed during the race. They consumed more than the recommended 60g carbohydrate per hour – the amount oxidized during high-intensity exercise – some going as high as 94g. They resorted to this high intake while riding because it was not practically possible to eat enough to meet their energy needs in the time available when not riding. The danger of a continued high intake of refined carbohydrates is that it can result in poor intakes of vitamins, especially the B vitamins.

As would be expected from sweat loss needs, fluid intake was high – an average of 6.7ℓ (14pt) per day – 4ℓ (8pt) of which was consumed while riding.

With so little time to recover before the next day's racing, these cyclists used enteral (tube feeds) formulae to supplement total energy, protein, fat and carbohydrate with additional micronutrient supplements.

Below *Tour de France cyclists need to consume a large percentage of their energy requirements while riding.*

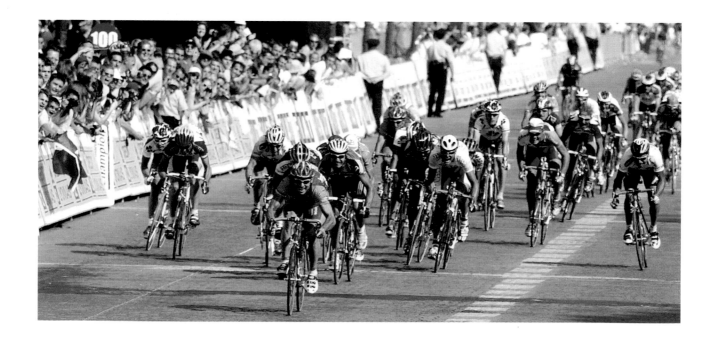

ALTITUDE

Nutritional requirements change at altitude – above 3500m (11,500ft). Acute Mountain Sickness (AMS) occurs within hours to three days after arrival at altitude. Symptoms include headache, nausea, vomiting and impaired thinking.

ENERGY

Exposure to altitudes above 3500m (11,500ft) increases Basal Metabolic Rate (BMR) by up to 28%, partly due to the extra effort of breathing. Decreased intake and increased expenditure of energy results in a deficit and weight loss of as much as 9kg (20 lb) during an expedition. Appetite is suppressed when you need it most. Energy intake should therefore be increased beyond appetite.

Energy deficit at high altitudes is also associated with negative protein balance and muscle wasting, therefore it is important to ensure a 12–20% protein intake. Because the total energy requirement during these events is so high the absolute amounts of carbohydrate, fat and protein are also high. Since fat is a more concentrated source of fuel, it makes practical sense to increase the total contribution of fat to the diet (*see case study on p175*).

FLUID

Extreme altitude exposure results in diuresis (increased flow of urine), with water and sodium losses, which increases the risk of dehydration during exercise. Fluid requirements are greater than at sea level and can be as high as 3–5ℓ (6–10pt) per day.

MICRONUTRIENTS

Altitude exposure is associated with increased oxidative stress (*see p89*) and many climbers use antioxidant supplements. The evidence for performance enhancement from these supplements is equivocal and there is also concern that these nutrients act as pro-oxidants if taken in high dosages for long periods. A multivitamin and antioxidant supplement would be more prudent.

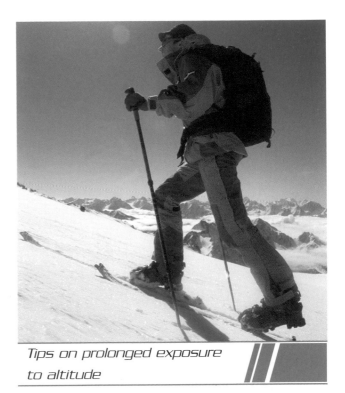

Tips on prolonged exposure to altitude

- Eat to plan, do not rely on an ad lib approach.
- Eat beyond normal satiety to diminish weight loss.
- Ensure adequate energy intakes as requirements are increased. However, due to the lower levels of daily activity the energy requirements will be less than expected.
- Drink at least 3–5ℓ (6–10pt) per day.
- Meet the Recommended Dietary Allowance (RDA) (*or RNI see p10*) for vitamins and minerals – you may need to use an antioxidant supplement containing vitamin C, E and alpha-lipoic acid.
- Ensure adequate iron stores prior to exposure.

Above *At altitude, appetite is suppressed when you need it most.*

PHYSICAL DEMANDS AND CHARACTERISTICS

ANTHROPOMETRY

In many of these activities a wider range of body size, shape and composition is acceptable, with higher body fat levels being an advantage (long distance open water swimming, for instance). In some events an athlete might even bulk up for the anticipated period of energy deficit (Everest, Trans-Atlantic row).

PHYSICAL DEMANDS

Every event has its own set of rules, many of which determine what and when you can eat. In the Ecochallenge you will only sleep for about two hours in 24, and a Trans-Atlantic row may have a two-hour-on, two-hour-off cycle. During an Ironman triathlon you can't eat while swimming or running.

ENVIRONMENT

The weather is uncontrollable and unpredictable. Temperatures can range from below freezing to above 50°C (122°F). In cold environments more energy is needed, whereas in hot environments dehydration is more likely to limit performance than lack of carbohydrate. An aggressive fluid plan is required during exercise and recovery, and will need to incorporate electrolytes.

COMMON NUTRITION ISSUES
INCREASED ENERGY NEEDS

Total energy needs for all these events is high and increased by carrying a heavy load (back pack, water and fluid). As the time spent exercising is prolonged, these calories cannot always be made up in the limited recovery time. If possible, weight changes should be monitored. Oils and fats can be used to boost calories. Snacks and fluids should be included as concentrated sources of energy. Protein requirements are sometimes difficult to achieve as many protein-rich foods are perishable and require more cooking compared to carbohydrate-rich quick-cooking noodles and sports bars.

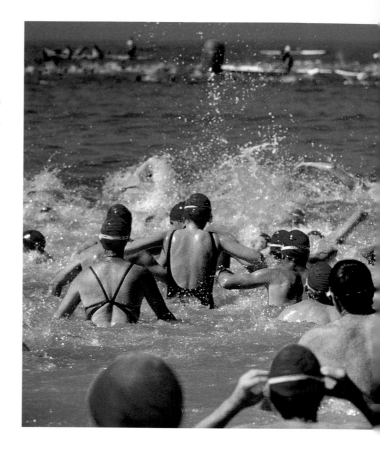

MUSCLE DAMAGE AND REPAIR

Exercise that results in muscle damage may also result in impaired glycogen synthesis and therefore recovery. This is partially overcome by increasing carbohydrate intake. Protein needs are also increased due to an increase in muscle and whole-body protein turnover, as well as increased oxidation of amino acids during and following exercise.

FLUID AND HYDRATION

Fluid losses are increased in hot enviroments and at altitude. Competitors face many practical obstacles to hydration such as faulty desalinators at sea, the time and effort required to melt snow at altitude, and access to and the weight of carrying water.

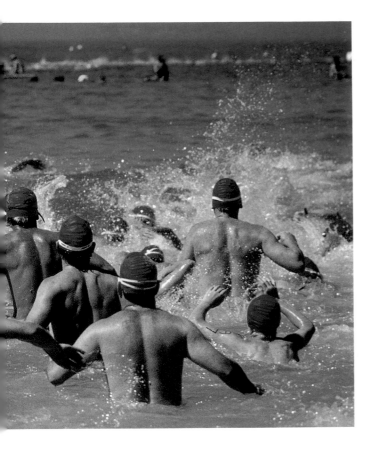

COMMON GAME PLAN – MULTIDAY EVENTS

A registered sports dietitian with specific experience in these events will give consideration to individuals within a team, teamwork, creative menus, the effective use of limited equipment, and contingency plans.

MEDICAL

Don't leave without having had a full medical and dental checkup. The nutrition first-aid kit should include the following preparatons:

- oral rehydration powder
- anti-nausea
- anti-diarrhoeal
- anti-motion sickness
- fibre/laxative

CREATIVE MENU PLANNING

To prevent 'menu fatigue,' work on a menu cycle. The plan must accommodate individual tastes and nutritional requirements (vegetarian, for instance) if part of a team event. Vary combinations, mix-and-match foods and include multiple flavours and herbs, but note that food and drinks may taste different during an event. Include treats for events such as birthdays and Christmas.

GENERAL ORGANIZATION

- When travelling, check out customs regulations with regard to bringing in food. Also investigate the option of purchasing familiar (safe) foods at your destination.
- You may want to send supplies to different ports or countries. This requires careful timing.
- When choosing foods, check the shelf life.
- Package and label foods clearly to prevent spoilage.
- Access to food during the event should allow for continuous 'grazing', by packing snacks in side pockets, for instance.
- Pack a reserve (you may incorporate freeze-dried food) as a back-up in case of weather delays and other unforeseen circumstances.

Above *Fuel availability, hydration, hyponatraemia and hunger are the nutritional challenges faced by triathletes.*

PORTABLE, LIGHTWEIGHT FOODS FOR MULTIDAY EVENTS

FOOD	PRACTICAL TIP
CARBOHYDRATE-RICH FOODS	
Rolled oats and instant cereals Breakfast cereals	Can also be enriched with extra skim milk powder and glucose polymer powders
Toasted muesli	Toasted is higher in fat and calories; for extra protein pre-mix with skim milk powder
Long-life bread	Useful for shorter events
Crackers and snack-bread	Can break and spoil easily; needs special packaging
Quick-cooking noodles and Ramen noodles Pasta and quick-cooking rice Quick-cooking pasta dishes	All require very little cooking
Couscous	Only needs boiling water; no cooking
Instant mashed potatoes	Saves time
Instant soups, thick	Good source of sodium
PROTEIN	
Beef jerky	Good source of protein, iron and sodium (salt)
Soya mince	–
Egg powder	–
Small cans of tuna, cooked meat, sardines	Heavy, but makes a nutritious change
Patés (e.g. goose liver)	–
Tuna sachets	Lighter option compared to tins
Instant/powdered cheese sauce	Can be added to vegetables and pasta dishes to boost protein
Cheese, cheese wedges	Can be included, depending on length of event and temperature
Parmesan cheese sachets	Adds flavour; better shelf life than other cheese
Salami and processed meats	Also a good source of fat; can be included for cooler climates, shorter trips
Pemmican	For emergencies and extreme expeditions
Dehydrated tofu	Can add to noodles, rice and vegetables – good option for vegetarians
Milk powder	Excellent source of protein, can be pre-mixed with cereals, added to drinks, soups
Liquid meal supplement powder	Can be used as a convenient light meal or snack or if appetite is lacking

FRUIT AND VEGETABLES	
Fresh fruit	You may be able to replenish stocks en route depending on event
Dried fruit	Compact and good source of energy and potassium
Dried fruit bars	–
Freeze-dried vegetables	–
Dehydrated vegetables	–
FATS	
Nuts	Mainly a source of fat, some protein. Caramelized and chocolate-coated adds calories
Seeds	–
Trail mix	–
Oil (olive)	Use to add calories (fat); olive oil adds flavour
CONFECTIONERY	
Chocolate bars	Not good in hot weather; soft chocolate squeezies in foil are better
Instant puddings, instant custard, chocolate mousse, Christmas pudding, panetonne, fruit cake	–
Sweets: nougat, jelly beans and jube sweets, wine gums	–
SPORTS-SPECIFIC PRODUCTS	
Sports drink powder	To boost carbohydrate and add electrolytes; adds flavour to water
Glucose polymer powders	Unflavoured carbohydrate boosters can be added to cereals and drinks
Sports bars and breakfast bars	Compact, energy dense
HOSPITALITY PACKS/INDIVIDUAL CATERING PACKS	
Salt, herbs, pepper, tomato sauce, ketchup, chutney, Worcestershire sauce, etc.	–
Tea bags, coffee, hot chocolate, cocoa, sugar sachets	–
Fruit cordial sachets	–
Fish spreads, yeast, vegetable and meat extract	–
Individual pesto sauces	–
Butter portions/nut butters/ peanut butter/jam	–
COMPLETE MEALS	
Freeze-dried instant meals	Compact vacuum-packed meals ready to eat (e.g. military meals), may be costly
Compact ready-to-eat meals	–

NUTRITION GAME PLAN SPECIFIC TO EVENTS

EVENT	SPECIFIC CHALLENGES	GAME PLAN
Ultra-marathon and Iron-man triathlon (4–13 hrs), e.g. Hawaiian Ironman Triathlon	Fuel availability (inadequate carbohydrate to sustain performance) Hydration Hyponatraemia Hunger	Fat-adapt and carbohydrate-load Provide 40–60g carbohydrate/hr during event choosing between solids and liquids depending on stage of event and appetite (e.g. easier to eat solids on the bike) Drink 400–800ml/hr (¾–1½pt/hr) depending on body weight, speed and temperature Ensure adequate electrolyte intakes via sports drinks, salt tablets, salty food When practical in the event, eat light, easily digestible carbohydrate-rich foods (e.g. sports bars, bananas, white bread jam sandwich, baby potatoes)
Multistage races (over several days/months; may involve different events), e.g. Tour de France Marathon des Sables; Raid Gauloises	Extreme energy needs; ongoing daily supply of adequate energy; limited recovery time Fluid Practical issues (food portage and preparation)	Make use of every opportunity to eat (e.g. if on the bike). Solid forms of carbohydrate may be eaten to prevent/alleviate hunger as well as continue to supply additional fuel Sports drinks with higher carbohydrate and electrolytes May be similar to Trans Ocean row – see below
Altitude expeditions, e.g. Everest; Patagonias	Altitude: ■ Acute mountain sickness (AMS) ■ Lack of appetite ■ Weight loss Fluid Antioxidants	Medication; small frequent meals Lightweight high-energy, high-nutrient dense foods *(select from Food Table pp178–179). If at special risk, try gaining weight beforehand; peer monitoring Fluid plan and 3–5ℓ (6–10pt) per day Cover your bases with a general antioxidant supplement There are some expeditions like Everest when during approach marches and at base camp you can rely on locally obtained foods, including a variety of fresh vegetables, potatoes, lentils, winter crops, rice, eggs, mutton and some fruit
Long distance swimming, e.g. English Channel, Florida Straits	Motion sickness Eating solids is difficult	Medication; ginger Sports drinks; gels; liquid meal replacements; soft foods (e.g. cream-filled sponge-cakes); pieces of sports bars; chocolate; soft cheese
Trans Ocean row e.g. Tenerife to Barbados Open water sailing, e.g. Cape to Rio; Whitbread	Time and difficulty in preparing food Weight of food Limited equipment Lack of fresh food High energy needs Fluid Motion sickness	Light, quick-cooking non-perishable nutrient-dense items (see p178–179). Always have stock of ready-to-eat meals when unable to prepare. Slow cooker (haybox); good-quality flask; quick shake; plastic bowls and cutlery (spares in case of rust or loss). Vitamin and mineral supplements Protein and carbohydrate powders; add oil to food; include high-fat snacks Water filters; iodine tablets; improve palatability of desalinated water by using flavoured carbohydrate powders Sea sickness can take up to five days; if necessary, take medication; ginger

CASE STUDY

EXTREME CUISINE

BACKGROUND

Ike McCarry* was joining two other climbers to ascend Mt McKinley in Alaska (6194m; 20,320ft). He wanted to avoid running out of food as they did on a previous adventure, in the Patagonias, when the weather turned bad. He also wanted to prevent excessive weight loss. On a previous expedition (at over 5000m; 16,400ft) he had lost 6kg (13 lb). His current weight was 85kg (187 lb).

* Name changed to protect client confidentiality.

DIETARY AND TRAINING HISTORY

He went to gym regularly (three to four hours per week). He would spend five hours per week walking on the mountain, carrying a 20kg (44 lb) load. He cycled 1–1½ hours once or twice a week.

RECOMMENDATIONS

GENERAL TIPS

His nutrition programme encompassed three phases:

1. Fat-loading regime
2. Carbohydrate-loading regime
3. A plan for the duration of the expedition

He was an engineer who enjoyed precision and numbers and was quite happy to be involved in the planning of his meals around the recommended calculations. He was also advised to establish a food and fluid plan in advance to ensure that he maintained an adequate energy and fluid intake of 3–5ℓ (6–10pt) per day. He chose a vitamin supplement which included 500mg vitamin C; 200–400 IU vitamin E; and 550mg alpha-lipoic acid.

Fat list	
EACH OF THE FOLLOWING PROVIDES 5G FAT	

5ml (1tsp) margarine, butter, oil or mayonnaise

10ml (2tsp) French salad dressing

20ml (4tsp) reduced-oil dressing

10ml (2tsp) peanut butter

¼ avocado pear

6 olives

1 rasher bacon

15ml (3tsp) sunflower/sesame seeds

2 walnuts

4 almonds

THREE DIETARY PHASES FOR AN ULTRA-ENDURANCE EVENT

	FAT-LOADING REGIME FIRST 5 DAYS (6–7 DAYS BEFORE EVENT)	CARBO-LOADING REGIME (2–3 DAYS BEFORE THE EVENT)	DURING EXPEDITION
ENERGY	17,422kJ (4168kcal)	16,649kJ (3964kcal)	16,720–18,810kJ (4000–4500kcal)
CARBOHYDRATE (G)	303 (29%)	650–700 (66%) 7–8g/kg	35% 350–400g minimum
PROTEIN (G)	145 (14%)	116 (12%)	150g (15%)
FAT (G)	264 (57%)	100 (22%)	222g (50%)

FAT-LOADING REGIME

	CARBOHYDRATE (G)	PROTEIN (G)	FAT (G)
BREAKFAST			
250ml (1 cup) toasted muesli	62	16	35
250ml (1 cup) full-cream milk	12	8	10
1 banana	15	–	–
12.5ml (1tbsp) sunflower seeds	–	2.7	6
8 almonds	–	3	8
Breakfast totals	89	30	59
SNACK			
100g (3⅓ oz) chocolate	60	9	31
LUNCH			
4 slices bread or 2 rolls or bagels	60	8	–
10ml (2tsp) margarine or ½ avocado	–	–	10
30ml (2tbsp) peanut butter	4	7	15
60g (2 oz) Cheddar cheese (2 matchboxes)	–	15	20
1 apple	15	–	–
(salad)	–	–	–
Lunch totals	79	30	45
SNACK			
250ml (1 cup) peanuts	18	28	80
25ml (2tbs) raisins	15	–	–
Snack totals	33	28	80
SUPPER			
125g (4 oz) chicken breast (roasted with skin) or fried meat or fish	–	36	14
250ml (1 cup) rice or pasta or 2 medium potatoes	30	4	–
salads/vegetables	–	–	–
25ml (2tbsp) French dressing or 20ml (4tsp) oil or 4 rashers bacon or 1 avocado	–	–	20
6 olives	–	–	5
250ml (1 cup) full-cream milk	12	8	10
salad	–	–	–
Supper totals	42	48	49
Daily totals	303g	145g	264g

On the expedition, where he was carrying all his supplies and did not want to rely on freeze-dried foods, the aim was to keep to a maximum of 1kg (2.2 lb) food per day.

MEALPLAN FOR THE EXPEDITION

BREAKFAST OPTIONS

FIRST OPTION

250ml (1 cup) toasted muesli

125ml (½ cup) full-cream milk powder

25ml (2tbsp) sunflower seeds

with the option of adding glucose polymer powder

SECOND OPTION

500ml (2 cups) high-fat liquid meal replacement

37.5ml (3tbsp) sunflower seeds

125ml (½ cup) chocolate-coated nuts

Total weight: 200–250g (0.44–0.55 lb)

Energy: 4276–5518kJ (1023–1320kcal)

Protein: 35g

Fat: 63g

Carbohydrate: 100g

LUNCH

6 high-fat biscuits/digestive biscuits

30ml (6tsp) butter

85g (3 oz) tuna or 60g (2 oz) cheese or 40g (1⅓ oz) beef jerky

72g (2½ oz) packet soup (optional)

Total weight: 300g (0.66 lb)

Energy: 5617kJ (1344kcal)

Protein: 34g

Fat: 75g

Carbohydrate: 142g

SNACKS

150g (5 oz) chocolate

125ml (½ cup) dried fruit

2 x 56g (2 oz) high-fat sports bars (30:40:30)

40g (1⅓ oz) glucose polymer powder

Total weight: 342g (0.75 lb)

Energy: aim for 6300kJ (1500kcal)

Protein: 40g

Fat: 60g

Carbohydrate: 210g

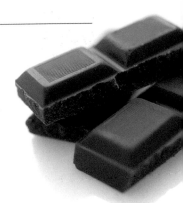

SUPPER EXAMPLE

170g (6 oz) tuna

85g (3 oz) noodles or 52g (2 oz) instant potato

5ml (1tsp) butter

25ml (2tbsp) malted food drink or cocoa

60ml (¼ cup) milk powder

Total weight: 300g (0.66 lb)

Energy: 4653kJ (1108kcal)

Protein: 43g

Fat 52g

Carbohydrate 78g

SOME OTHER IDEAS

- For suppers, he was advised to purchase ready meals or combinations of foods.
- Couscous was suggested as a carbohydrate option because it is light and very quick to cook, requiring little water. For taste he could add sun-dried tomatoes in oil with olives and grated cheese.
- Pesto sauce with pasta and Parmesan. He could have this with salami or beef jerky for extra protein or a high-fat liquid meal replacement.

Left *The fat-loading regime was started seven days before the start of the expedition.*

CARBOHYDRATE-LOADING EATING PLAN

BREAKFAST	
50g carbohydrate	375ml (1½ cup) breakfast cereal and low-fat milk
1 fruit	1 banana
25g carbohydrate	250ml (8 fl oz) fruit juice
MID-MORNING	
50g carbohydrate	2 slices of bread and 12.5ml (1tbsp) jam
2 fats	20ml (4tsp) peanut butter
50g carbohydrate	40ml (3½tbsp) raisins
LUNCH	
50g carbohydrate	3 medium potatoes or 375ml (1½ cup) rice
2 proteins	70g (2⅓ oz) lean meat or 80g (3 oz) chicken or 100g (3⅓ oz) fish
3 fats	5ml (1tsp) oil or margarine and ½ avocado (for salad)
Vegetables	vegetables/salad
25g carbohydrate	250ml (8 fl oz) fruit juice
SNACK	
50g carbohydrate	250ml (1 cup) fruit yoghurt
1 fruit	1 peach
50g carbohydrate	9 jelly babies
SUPPER	
50g carbohydrate	375ml (1½ cup) rice or 250–500ml (1–2 cups) pasta or 2 large rolls
5 proteins	175g (6 oz) meat or 200g (7 oz) chicken or 250g (8 oz) fish
3 fats	6 olives, 10ml (2tsp) French dressing and 5ml (1tsp) oil for food preparation (*see Fat List p175*)
Vegetables	vegetables/salads
1 fruit	1 orange
EXTRA	
100g carbohydrate	1.25–1.5ℓ (2½–3pt) sports drink
50g carbohydrate	500–600ml (17–20 fl oz) Coke during the day
50g carbohydrate	60ml (12tsp sugar) with cereal or coffee
25g carbohydrate	500–750ml (2–3 cups) low-fat milk with cereal or coffee

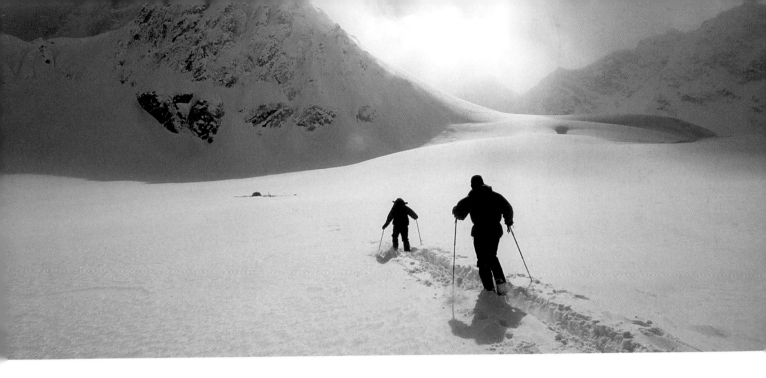

FROM THE MEMOIRS OF McCARRY

'The first five or six days I believe I kept approximately to the suggested calories and the carbohydrate, fat and protein split. With altitude (above 3500m; 11,500ft), once again, the desire to eat fell off. I did start off with much enthusiasm to keep a record of intake but the snowstorm became a bit of a survival thing and I became distracted and never got a real grip again on writing down the details.

We communally ate dehydrated food for breakfast and dinner – three-bean chilli became a hot favourite. For lunch we each took our own. For me: salami, beef jerky, Stilton cheese, butter, tortillas, chocolate bars and nuts and raisins.

A snowstorm locked us in on the lower glacier for two days, but after that – relatively fine weather. We were always pushing to beat the next potential storm. Sadly my two colleagues fell apart mentally somewhat before high camp and needed severe coercion. It meant I soloed the summit, which of course became a personal ethereal adventure that will never be forgotten.

By the eighth day, and high camp at 5250m (17,225ft), I was forcing down food. The ninth day was summit day and I was undernourished, and I knew it. On a large expansive snowfield before the summit ridge, on the way up, I almost collapsed from exhaustion – I had two chocolate bars and felt better after 15 minutes. The same thing happened on the way back – too tired to move – ate my last chocolate bar and forced on. Halfway down the summit ridge I tripped and fell, simply because I was exhausted. I knew before I left camp I didn't have enough food inside me from the dinner the previous evening and the morning breakfast, but still I went ahead and climbed – mentally very, very focused and determined. I really must watch that situation next time. Waterwise, I insisted everyone drink a minimum of 3ℓ (6pt) a day. The cold dry air sucks out large quantities of moisture just from breathing and by 4500m (14,765ft), breathing is rapid with strenuous activity. For me I had three or four cups of tea or cocoa at breakfast, similar for dinner, plus soup, and carried one 1ℓ (2pt) bottle with me when climbing. I found this was sufficient.'

Above *Fluid requirements are increased at altitude – above 3500m (11,500ft).*
Opposite *McCarry was given a 50g carbohydrate list (see p17) from which to select and create his own menus.*

glossary

Adipose tissue An aggregation of fat cells (adipocytes) containing large reserves of fat – providing both insulation and an energy reserve.

Adenosine diphosphate (ADP) The high-energy compound formed when one phosphate group is split from ATP in the process of releasing energy.

Adenosine triphosphate (ATP) a nucleotide consisting of a sugar base (adenosine) and three high energy phosphate groups which are broken down during metabolism, releasing energy for important physiological processes.

Aerobic Process requiring oxygen. Fat can only provide energy in the presence of oxygen (aerobic lipolysis). Carbohydrate can be used to fuel exercise with (aerobic glycolysis) or without oxygen (anaerobic glycolysis).

Aerobic exercise refers to an activity that increases your pulse rate and places demands on your cardiovascular system and, over time, produces beneficial changes in your respiratory and circulatory systems.

Alpha-amylase An enzyme, secreted by the salivary glands, that breaks down carbohydrate.

Amenorrhea The complete cessation of normal menstrual function/flow as a result of hormonal changes – often associated with reduced food intake and low body weight.

Amino acids function as the building blocks of proteins. There are 22 different amino acids. There are nine essential amino acids, so-called because they are not manufactured by the body and must come from the diet.

Anabolic The synthesis of new material – compounds or tissue – the opposite of catabolic.

Anaemia A deficiency in haemoglobin, red blood cells, or packed cell volume (*see entry*) and thus oxygen uptake, transportation and utilization may be impaired. Most anaemias are caused by a lack of nutrients required for red blood cell synthesis – principally iron, vitamin B_{12}, and folic acid.

Anaerobic Without the use of oxygen.

Anthropometry The science of measuring the size, weight, and proportions of the human body.

Antioxidant A substance (e.g. vitamins C and E) that can inhibit the damage caused by free radicals which are formed in the body as a result of oxidative stress (see entry) such as excessive exposure to environmental pollution, ultraviolet light, illness or cigarette smoke.

ATP see Adenosine triphosphate

Basal metabolism The energy (kilojoules/calories) a body burns when completely at rest to keep involuntary body processes going (processes include heartbeat, breathing, generating body heat, perspiring to keep cool, and transmitting messages to the brain).

Bone densitometry Measurement of bone using tissue absorption of x-rays (photons) by an instrument called a dual energy x-radiographic absorptiometer (DXA).

Buffer A substance or solution which can prevent rapid changes in the concentrations of a given ion and pH.

Calorie (also kilocalorie – kcal) The traditional unit of energy (*see also conversions p8*) 1 kilojoule≈4.184 kcal.

Carnitine Synthesized in the human liver and kidney from the essential amino acids methionine and lysine. Facilitates the use of long-chain fatty acids as an energy source. Carnitine supplements do not appear to increase levels of carnitine in the muscle.

Carotenaemia A condition resulting from continued high intakes of beta carotene in which the skin takes on a yellow tinge, particularly on the palms of the hands and the soles of the feet. This is not harmful, and the skin slowly returns to its normal colour when carotenoid intake is reduced.

Carbohydrate glucose polymer powders Carbohydrate powders with a bland taste formed by splitting large starch molecules into glucose chains of, usually, 7–10 units.

Carbo-loading Increasing the glycogen reserves in skeletal muscle by a combination of diet (consuming up to 8–10g carbohydrate per kg bodyweight) and an exercise taper.

Catabolic Break-down of tissue or compounds – the opposite of anabolic.

Couscous A cereal processed from semolina into tiny pellets, best known for its use in the traditional North African dish of that name.

Creatine phosphokinase (CPK) is a catalyst in the processes of storing energy (PCr (CP) + ADP) and releasing energy (Cr + ATP).

Creatine phosphate (CP) (Also Phosphocreatine – PCr) a limited, but rapidly available, source of fuel that regenerates ATP within the muscle tissue, which provides energy.

Dietary fibre The indigestible portion of plant materials such as cellulose, lignin, pectin and gums.

Dietary Reference Intakes (DRIs) The universally accepted set of nutrient-based reference values used to assess and plan diets. This includes reference values used for individuals such as the RDAs (gender-specific recommended dietary allowances for various stages of life) and ULs (upper tolerance/safe levels). Nutrient intakes beyond the UL may increase rather than reduce health risks.

Dietary Reference Values (DRVs) Used in the United Kingdom, the generic term for Estimated Average Requirement (EAR), Reference Nutrient Intake (RNI) and Lower Reference Nutrient Intake (LRNI).

Diuresis Increased secretion of urine.

Dysmenorrhea The disturbance of normal menstrual function, often temporary.

Electrolytes Minerals (such as sodium, potassium, magnesium and calcium) that circulate in the body fluids and help to regulate the body's fluid balance. Small amounts are lost in sweat and need to be replaced either by electrolyte-containing sports drinks or food.

Enzyme Complex protein molecules that act as biological catalysts – increase the rate of a chemical reaction without itself being changed at the end of the reaction.

Ergogenic aids Performance enhancers, from the Greek words *ergon* meaning work, and *-genic*, relating to production or generation.

Fatty acids The structural components of fats.

Free radicals Highly reactive substances that result from exposure to oxygen, background radiation, and other environmental factors. They cause cellular damage in the body, which can be repaired by antioxidants.

Fructose The monosaccharide found in fruit, honey and some vegetables; also obtained from the hydrolysis of sucrose (sucrose = glucose + fructose).

Gluconeogenesis The production of new glucose, not from glycogen, but from other metabolites such as amino acids and fatty acids when blood sugar levels drop (during fasting and starvation).

Glutamine A nonessential amino acid that can be synthesized by various tissues such as the skeletal muscles, liver, and fat. Various cells of the immune system such as the lymphocytes and macrophages depend on glutamine as a primary fuel source. During exercise (or other times of metabolic stress – fasting, severe injury, illness), the demand for plasma glutamine increases.

Glycaemic Index (GI) A ranking of the effect on blood glucose level of the consumption of a single food, relative to a reference carbohydrate (e.g. white bread or glucose).

Glycaemic Load Whereas GI determines the rate of a food's effect on blood glucose levels, the glycaemic load also considers the amount of carbohydrate eaten.

Glycogen The storage form of glucose in animal cells, mainly liver and skeletal muscle.

Glycolysis The breaking down of glucose into simpler compounds, chiefly pyruvate or lactate.

Homocysteine An amino acid produced in the human body. It is usually chemically transformed into methionine and cysteine with the help of folic acid and vitamins B_{12}, and B_6. Insufficient B_{12}, and B_6 can hamper the breakdown of homocysteine, causing it to accumulate in the blood, which is a risk factor for coronary heart disease.

Hypoglycaemia A deficiency of sugar in the blood caused by too much insulin or too little glucose.

Insulin A hormone secreted by the pancreas that helps regulate carbohydrate metabolism.

Hyponatraemia Low sodium levels in the blood.

Hypothermic Lower than normal body temperature.

Hypotonic Solutions with osmotic pressures lower than that of the solution to which it is compared (usually body fluids) thus causing a net flow of water across the semi-permeable cell membrane into the cell.

Hyperglycaemia Greater than normal levels of glucose in the blood.

Hypertonic Solutions with osmotic pressures greater than that of the solution to which it is compared (usually body fluids) thus causing a net flow of water across the semi-permeable cell membrane out of the cell.

Hyperthermic Greater than normal body temperature.

Immunoglobulin A (IgA) Protects against infections. It is secreted by the bowel and upper respiratory mucosa.

Immunoglobulin E (IgE) The antibody in the immune system that reacts with allergens.

Immunosuppression The prevention or reduction in immune response caused by, for example, irradiation, antibodies, viral infection or specific chemical agents.

Isotonic Equal osmotic pressure between two solutions.

Kilojoules (kJ) The basic units in which the energy value of food and the energy needs of the body are measured. 1 kJ≈4.184 kcal (referred to simply as calories).

Lactate/lactic acid A product of glycolysis, formed when the rate of pyruvate production exceeds pyruvate oxidation and rapidly dissociates into lactate and hydrogen ions. It is produced and used by the muscles as a fuel.

Lanugo Fine downy hair on the body, which may be a feature of anorexia nervosa.

Lean body mass (LBM) The total of all body components except fat and bone.

Leptin (Greek *leptos*, meaning thin.) A protein hormone which helps regulate body weight, metabolism and reproduction.

Lymphocytes White blood cells involved in the immune system – B cells and T cells.

Lysosomes Structures of cell cytoplasm that contain digestive enzymes.

Lysozyme An enzyme in saliva, tears, egg white and other animal fluids, which can break down bacterial cell walls.

Macrophages Large cells distributed through the body that play a major role in immune defence.

Macronutrients Nutrients needed in relatively large amounts for energy – carbohydrates, proteins and fats.

Metabolism The chemical and physiological processes by which the body builds and maintains itself and breaks down food and nutrients for energy.

Micronutrients Nutrients such as vitamins and minerals essential to health, but needed in very small amounts.

Muscle fibre types Type I (slow-twitch) muscle fibres have an increased capacity to produce ATP by oxygen-dependent metabolism in the mitochondria. Long-distance runners and cross-country skiers have a high percentage of Type I fibres. Type II (fast-twitch) muscle fibres have a low mitochondrial content and contract rapidly. Sprinters, jumpers and weight lifters have a high percentage of Type II fibres

Neuro-protection Protects the nervous system.

Nutraceutical/Functional food Any substance in food which is specifically developed with claimed health benefits.

Osmolality A measure of the osmotically active particles per kg of solvent in which the particles are dissolved and is expressed as mOsm/kg.

Osmolarity A measure of the osmotically active particles per litre of solution and is expressed as mmol/ℓ

Osteopenia Too little bone mass at any stage of the life cycle; a specific definition of bone conditions that is based on bone densitometry.

Osteoporosis Loss of bone tissue to the point of being unable to sustain ordinary strains. Diagnosis based on bone density measurement.

Oxidation The process of releasing energy from nutrients. A process undergoing a chemical reaction with oxygen.

Oxidative stress Free radicals (products of normal cell processes) wreak havoc in their hunt for a mate. The oxygen molecule's unpaired electron makes it unstable and electrically charged. It stabilizes by interacting with the nearest available molecule, targeting fats, proteins and DNA. Free radicals' actions can damage molecules and kill cells.

Packed cell volume The ratio of the volume occupied by packed red blood cells to the volume of the whole blood.

Periodization (in sport) Training based on the manipulation of volume (how much) and intensity (how hard) of the work done during different phases of the season. A dietary regime can be periodized to meet the requirements of training and competition.

Phospho-creatine (PCr) See creatine phosphate (CP).

Phosphate A salt of phosphoric acid. Inorganic phosphate can be formed by the reactions of ATP or ADP with the formation of the corresponding ADP or AMP and the release of a phosphate ion.

Placebo Sometimes casually referred to as a 'sugar pill,' a placebo is a 'fake' treatment which seems identical to the real treatment. Placebo treatments are used to eliminate bias that may arise from the expectation that a treatment should produce an effect.

Plant sterols and stanols A component in wood oils, corn, soy and wheat which may reduce the risk of coronary heart disease by lowering blood cholesterol levels.

Polenta A type of meal ground from sweetcorn or maize.

Postural hypotension A drop in blood pressure (hypotension) due to a change in body position (posture) when sitting up or standing up. A temporary reduction in blood flow, and therefore a shortage of oxygen to the brain, causes lightheadedness and sometimes a 'black out'.

Prebiotics Non-digestible food products that stimulate the growth of symbiotic bacterial species already present in the colon; they help improve health.

Proanthocyanidins A type of tannin found in cranberries, cocoa and chocolate which may improve urinary tract health and reduce the risk of cardiovascular disease.

Probiotics Microbial foods or supplements that can change or re-establish the intestinal flora and improve health.

Quorn A mycoprotein (and related to mushrooms, truffles, and morel). Nutritious and has a meat-like texture.

Samp Dry maize kernels pounded or stamped until broken, but not as fine as mealie meal. Samp is prepared and cooked in the same way as dried beans – and served with a lump of butter or fat.

Sports anaemia A transient anaemia seen in heavily training athletes. A decrease in the red blood cell count, haemoglobin concentration, and packed cell volume, but with normal red cell morphology.

Stress Fractures A break in a bone, usually small, that develops because of repeated or prolonged forces.

Stressor An agent, condition, or other stimulus that causes stress to an organism.

Teratogenic Substances that can interfere with normal embryonic development and non-heritable birth defects.

Thermic effect of food Increased energy expenditure due to the amount of energy spent in the metabolic process of digestion, breakdown and storage of food.

Thiol antioxidants Sulfur-containing phytonutrients (found in e.g. broccoli, cauliflower, brussel sprouts, kale and cabbage) that upregulate enzymes involved in the detoxification of carcinogens and other foreign compounds.

Thyroid hormones Modulate tissue responsiveness to catecholamines (stress hormones) secreted by the Sympathetic Nervous System (SNS). Levels of these hormones determine adapative thermogenesis. Subtle defects may predispose some to excessive weight gain.

Trans fats Occur naturally in beef, butter, milk and lamb fats and in commercially prepared, partially hydrogenated margarines and solid cooking fats. However, trans fats, like saturated fats, raise blood LDL cholesterol levels (the 'bad' cholesterol). High consumption of trans fats may also reduce the HDL or 'good' cholesterol levels.

VO_2 max A measure of maximal oxygen uptake; litres of oxygen consumed per kilogram of body weight per minute.

index

Bold numbers indicate an illustration on that page.

macrophages 88

magic claims for supplements *104*

magnesium 103, 104

ma huang 96, 100

make weight (see also weight-making) 60, 62

master athletes 42–43

  nutritional needs of 43

MCTs 166, 102

meal planning 46–48

measurements 10–11

medium chain triglycerides (MCT oils) 166

menarche 33

menstrual

  disturbances 117

  dysfunction 33, 75, 76, 77

menu planning 171

metabolism 110

methylguanidine acetic acid (*see also under creatine*) 97

micronutirients and chronic fatigue 91

micronutrient (*see also vitamins and minerals*) 22, 24, 88, 89, 91

  food sources of 24

  requirements at altitude 169

  requirements of children 35

multiday events, portable, light-weight food for 172–173 172

muscle damage 14, 22, 39

  and repair 170

muscle dysmorphia 78

muscle fibre type 149

muscle glycogen 148, 150

muscle mass, increased 97, 98, 99

Nandrolone 94, 96, 104, 105

nandrolone precursor steroid 105

National Collegiate Athletic Association 117

nausea 65, 67

Newby Fraser, Paula 30

nor-pseudoephedrine 100

nutraceuticals 90

nutrient properties, comparison of 132

nutrition

  as component of performance *14*

  needs of children 35

  status 117

Oligomenorrhoea 76

Ornish, Dean (weight-loss diet) 129, 130

osmolality 65, 66

osmolality of blood 66

osteoporosis 76, 117, 126

overhydration 65

  signs of 65

oxidative stress 42, 89, 169

Palatability 65, 68

perceived exertion 116

perception of effort 13, 14, 30, 61

performance enhancing 13

phenylalanine 98

phosphagen 148

phospho creatine (PCr) 97

Physical Activity Levels (PAL) 35

phytochemicals 90

phyto-oestrogens 103

plant sterols 90

plate model **23**

polyunsaturated fats 20

pre-competition nutrition 52

pre-competition snacks 53

pregnancy and lactation 40–41

  exercise during 41

Pritikin (weight-loss diet) 129

proanthrocyanidins 90

product purity 143

profile of mood states (POMS) 116

prohormones 104

ACKNOWLEDGEMENTS

We would like to thank and acknowledge our friends and colleagues at the Sports Science Institute of South Africa who have supported us in the preparation of *Eating for Sport*. The assistance of staff from the High Performance Unit and Professors Mike and Vicki Lambert from the UCT/MRC Research Unit for Exercise Science and Sports Medicine was especially appreciated.

We would also like to express our gratitude to all the teams and athletes with whom we have worked over the years. This has provided us with much practical insight.

Thanks also to the staff at New Holland Publishers – Alfred LeMaitre, who commissioned the book, our editor Anna Tanneberger for her expert advice and patience, and Nathalie Scott and Steven Felmore for their creative design and illustrations.

PHOTOGRAPHIC CREDITS

Copyright rests with the following photographers and/or their agents listed below.
Key to Locations: t = top; b = bottom; l = left; r = right; c = centre.
NHIL...New Holland Image Library / A = André Wepener, MC = Michael Cowell, M = Micky Hoyle, N = Nicholas Aldridge,
P = Pieter Smit, R = Ryno Reyneke, W = Warren Heath.
IOA...Images of Africa / A = Anthony Johnson, D = Dirk Pieters, DB = Dominic Barnardt, J = Jacques Marais, JP = John Peacock
K = Kelly Walsh, M = Mark Skinner, RD= Roger de la Harpe, R = Ryno Reyneke, S = Shaen Adey

Front cover	t	NHIL/N		38	c	IOA/K		80–81		Photo Access	
Front cover – middle row (from left to right): Photo Access, IOA/D, Tim de Frisco, NHIL/R, Photo Access				38	b	IOA/R		86		Photo Access	
				39	t	IOA/D		87		NHIL/R	
				39	c	NHIL/A		88		NHIL/M	
Front cover	bl	Photo Access		39	b	NHIL/W		89		NHIL/W	
Front cover	br	NHIL/R		40		NHIL/R		90		NHIL/A	
Back cover	t	NHIL/R		41		NHIL/W		92–93		NHIL/N	
Back cover	c	IOA/J		42	tl	NHIL/R		94		NHIL/W	
Back cover	b	NHIL/R		42	r	Photo Access		95	tl	NHIL/R	
Front flap	t	Photo Access		43	tl	NHIL/W		95	br	NHIL/A	
Front flap	b	NHIL/R		43	br	NHIL/R		96–97		NHIL/N	
Back flap		IOA/R		44–45		Photo Access		99		NHIL/N	
2–3		NHIL/N		47		NHIL/R		100		NHIL/A	
4–5		Photo Access		52	tl	IOA		106		Digital Source	
6–7		NHIL/N		52	tr	NHIL/A		108–109		NHIL/R	
8–9		NHIL/N		53		NHIL/A		111	tr	IOA/S	
10		IOA/R		54		Sporting Pictures (UK)		111	bl	Photo Access	
11		NHIL/A		55		Photo Access		112	l	NHIL/R	
12–13		Photo Access		56		NHIL/A		112	r	NHIL/P	
15		NHIL/R		57		NHIL/W		113		NHIL/MC	
18	l	IOA/A		58–59		Photo Access		114	tl	NHIL/N	
18	r	Photo Access		60–61		Victah Sailor/Photo Run		114	tr	NHIL/R	
21		IOA/A		62		NHIL/W		115	tr	Action Images/Paul Gilham/Photo Access	
24		IOA/A		64		NHIL/N		115	bl	NHIL/N	
26		NHIL/W		65		IOA/J		116		NHIL/N	
28		NHIL/R		66		NHIL/R		119	l	IOA/JP	
31		Touchline		68	t	NHIL/R		119	r	NHIL/R	
32–33		Photo Access		68	tr	NHIL/R		120		Photo Access	
34		Photo Access		69	r	IOA/K		121		NHIL/R	
35		NHIL/W		70–71		Photo Access		122		IOA/S	
36		Photo Access		73		Tim de Frisco		123	l	NHIL/A	
37	t	NHIL/R		75		Photo Access		123	r	NHIL/W	
37	c	NHIL/R		77		Sporting Pictures/Greg Crisp		124–125		IOA/DB	
37	b	Photo Access		79		NHIL/N		127		NHIL/N	
38	t	IOA/C									

128		Photo Access
130		NHIL/A
131		NHIL/W
134		NHIL/A
136		Action Images/Brandon Malone/Photo Access
138		Gallo Images/gettyimages.com
140		Touchline
142		Photo Access
143		IOA/A
144		NHIL/A
146–147		NHIL/N
148		NHIL/N
149		Tim de Frisco
150–151		All Sport USA/Mike Powell
153		NHIL/W
154–155		Photo Access
159		NHIL/A
160		PPL
161		NHIL/R
162–163		IOA/RD
165	t	Tim de Frisco
165	br	NHIL/R
166		Touchline
167	t	NHIL/R
167	c	IOA/J
167	b	IOA/M
168		Action Images/Tom Able – Green Digital/Photo Access
169		Photo Access
170–171		Photo Access
177		NHIL/R
179		Photo Access

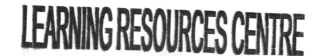